Beyond Loss

Beyond Loss

DEMENTIA, IDENTITY, PERSONHOOD

EDITED BY LARS-CHRISTER HYDÉN,
HILDE LINDEMANN,
and
JENS BROCKMEIER

OXFORD
UNIVERSITY PRESS

OXFORD
UNIVERSITY PRESS

Oxford University Press is a department of the University of
Oxford. It furthers the University's objective of excellence in research,
scholarship, and education by publishing worldwide.

Oxford New York
Auckland Cape Town Dar es Salaam Hong Kong Karachi
Kuala Lumpur Madrid Melbourne Mexico City Nairobi
New Delhi Shanghai Taipei Toronto

With offices in
Argentina Austria Brazil Chile Czech Republic France Greece
Guatemala Hungary Italy Japan Poland Portugal Singapore
South Korea Switzerland Thailand Turkey Ukraine Vietnam

Oxford is a registered trademark of Oxford University Press
in the UK and certain other countries.

Published in the United States of America by
Oxford University Press
198 Madison Avenue, New York, NY 10016

© Oxford University Press 2014

All rights reserved. No part of this publication may be reproduced, stored in
a retrieval system, or transmitted, in any form or by any means, without the prior
permission in writing of Oxford University Press, or as expressly permitted by law,
by license, or under terms agreed with the appropriate reproduction rights organization.
Inquiries concerning reproduction outside the scope of the above should be sent to the
Rights Department, Oxford University Press, at the address above.

You must not circulate this work in any other form
and you must impose this same condition on any acquirer.

Library of Congress Cataloging-in-Publication Data
Beyond loss : dementia, identity, personhood / edited by Lars-Christer Hydén, Hilde Lindemann,
and Jens Brockmeier.
    p. ; cm.
Includes bibliographical references.
ISBN 978–0–19–996926–5 (alk. paper)
I. Hydén, Lars-Christer, 1954– editor of compilation.   II. Lindemann, Hilde, editor of compilation.
III. Brockmeier, Jens, editor of compilation.
[DNLM: 1. Dementia. 2. Alzheimer Disease. 3. Personhood. WM 220]
RC521
616.8′3—dc23
2013036140

9 8 7 6 5 4 3 2 1
Printed in the United States of America
on acid-free paper

Contents

List of Contributors   vii

Introduction: Beyond Loss: Dementia, Identity, Personhood   1
   LARS-CHRISTER HYDÉN, HILDE LINDEMANN, AND JENS BROCKMEIER

Part One   PERSONS, PERSONHOOD, AND DIGNITY

1. Second Nature and the Tragedy of Alzheimer's   11
   HILDE LINDEMANN

2. The Person with Dementia as Understood through Stern's Critical Personalism   24
   STEVEN R. SABAT

3. Dignity and Dementia: A Conceptual Exploration   39
   LENNART NORDENFELT

4. "I'm his wife not his carer!"—Dignity and Couplehood in Dementia   53
   INGRID HELLSTRÖM

Part Two   IDENTITY, AGENCY, EMBODIMENT

5. Questions of Meaning: Memory, Dementia, and the Postautobiographical Perspective   69
   JENS BROCKMEIER

6. Everyday Dramas: Comparing Life with Dementia
   and Acquired Brain Injury   91
   MARIA I. MEDVED

7. Musical Embodiment, Selfhood, and Dementia   107
   PIA C. KONTOS

8. As the Body Speaks: Creative Expression in Dementia   120
   ALISON PHINNEY

Part Three   COMMUNICATION, FAMILY, AND INSTITUTIONS

9. How to Do Things with Others: Joint Activities Involving
   Persons with Alzheimer's Disease   137
   LARS-CHRISTER HYDÉN

10. Comprehension in Interaction: Communication at
    a Day-care Center   155
    CAMILLA LINDHOLM

11. "Familyhood" and Young-onset Dementia: Using Narrative and
    Biography to Understand Longitudinal Adjustment to
    Diagnosis   173
    PAMELA ROACH, JOHN KEADY, AND PENNY BEE

12. The Subjectivity of Disorientation: Moral Stakes
    and Concerns   191
    LINDA ÖRULV

Index   209

List of Contributors

Penny Bee is a Senior Lecturer & Health Services Researcher within the School of Nursing, Midwifery & Social Work, University of Manchester. Penny research interests focus on understanding concepts of health and healthcare provision from service user and carer perspectives, predominantly within the context of mental health. Over the last decade, Penny has conducted many local, regional and national studies evaluating the implementation of more accessible ways of delivering mental health services, with a key emphasis on service re-design to enhance service user and carer support.

Jens Brockmeier, a Professor at the American University of Paris, has a background in psychology, philosophy, and language studies. His interests are in issues of memory, identity, and the autobiographical process, which he has examined in a variety of cultural contexts and languages and under conditions of health and illness.

Ingrid Hellström has a PhD in caring sciences, especially in ageing and later life from Linköping University, Sweden, and is Associate Professor in palliative care at Ersta Sköndal University College, Sweden. She has a position as Senior Lecturer at the Department of Social and Welfare Studies and Researcher at the Center for Dementia Research at Linköping University. As a registered nurse she has several years experience of working with people with dementia and their families in different stages of the disease.

Lars-Christer Hydén received his PhD in psychology from Stockholm University, Sweden. His current position is as full Professor of Social Psychology at Linköping University, Sweden, and as Director of Center for Dementia Research. His research primarily concerns how people with Alzheimer's disease and their significant others interact and use language—especially narrative—as a way to sustain and negotiate identity and a sense of self.

John Keady is a registered mental health nurse and completed his part-time PhD in 1999. Since 2006 John has worked at The University of Manchester, England where he holds a joint Professorial position between the School of Nursing, Midwifery and Social Work and the Greater Manchester West Mental Health NHS Foundation Trust. John currently leads the inter-disciplinary Dementia and Ageing Research Team and he is founding and co-editor of the bi-monthly Sage journal. Dementia: the international journal of social research and practice; first edition published 2002.

Pia C. Kontos is a Senior Research Scientist at Toronto Rehabilitation Institute-University Health Network, Toronto, Canada, and Associate Professor at the Dalla Lana School of Public Health, University of Toronto. Her academic training is in medical anthropology, gerontology, and public health sciences. Central to her program of research is "embodied selfhood," a philosophy and approach to person-centered care that emphasizes the importance of the body for self-expression. Her research relies heavily on arts-based methodologies both as a strategy for implementing embodied selfhood into practice and for their creative and innovative potential to engage persons with dementia in meaningful ways. She has presented and published across multiple disciplines.

Hilde Lindemann is a Professor of Philosophy at Michigan State University. A former president of the American Society for Bioethics and Humanities and a Fellow of the Hastings Center, her published work includes *Damaged Identities, Narrative Repair; An Invitation to Feminist Ethics*; and *Holding and Letting Go: The Social Practice of Personal Identities*. She edited *Stories and Their Limits: Narrative Approaches to Bioethics* and coedited *Naturalized Bioethics: Toward Responsible Knowing and Practice*.

Camilla Lindholm is an Academy Research Fellow in Scandinavian Studies at the University of Helsinki, Finland. Lindholm uses the methods of conversation analysis and interactional linguistics to investigate interaction in institutional settings and conversations involving participants with communication difficulties. Her current research interests involve communication interventions and multilingual encounters in dementia care.

Maria I. Medved is an Associate Professor in the Department of Psychology at the University of Manitoba, Winnipeg, Canada. She is also a licensed psychologist who practices in clinical psychology, neuropsychology, and rehabilitation psychology. Her research is concerned with the way people deal with threats to their self-identity in disease or after injury. Her research is concerned with people as they go through a particular kind of developmental crisis, a crisis of self or identity due to injury or disease.

Lennart Nordenfelt is since 1987 Professor of Philosophy of Medicine and Health Care at the Department of Medical and Health Sciences, University of

Linköping, Sweden. He became Professor at the transdisciplinary faculty of themes at Linköping University in 1987. He initiated there a research program under the title Theory, Ethics and Ideology of Health Care. Nordenfelt's monographs include *On the Nature of Health* (1995), *Rationality and Compulsion* (2007), and *Dignity in the Care for Older People* (2009). He was Visiting Professor at the University of Warwick, England, in 1998–1999. Nordenfelt was between 2001 and 2004 President of the European Society for the Philosophy of Medicine and Health Care.

Alison Phinney is an Associate Professor at the University of British Columbia School of Nursing in Vancouver, Canada, and a Research Associate of the Centre for Research on Personhood in Dementia. She has long been interested in how it is for people to live with dementia, most recently focusing on the practical question of how to best support meaningful activity for people in the earlier stages of the disease. Throughout this work, she has drawn on phenomenological traditions in nursing to uncover experiences of the lived body, with an aim to better understand questions of identity and meaning.

Pamela Roach is currently a Postdoctoral Research Fellow with the Department of Family Medicine at the University of Alberta in Edmonton, Canada. She has a background in physical anthropology from the University of Calgary and completed her PhD at the University of Manchester in Manchester, England. She has experience working in mental health research in both the Canadian and UK health care systems and her primary research foci include family relationships, young-onset dementia, and qualitative research methods.

Steven R. Sabat is Professor of Psychology at Georgetown University, Washington, DC. The focus of his research, published in numerous scientific journal articles, has been on the intact cognitive and social abilities and the subjective experience of people with moderate to severe dementia, as well as on how to enhance communication between people with dementia and their carers. He is also the author of *The Experience of Alzheimer's Disease: Life through a Tangled Veil* and coeditor of *Dementia: Mind, Meaning, and the Person*.

Linda Örulv, PhD, is a team member of the Center for Dementia Research, Linköping University, Sweden. Her thesis focused on how residents in dementia care units actively and creatively used their remaining linguistic and cognitive resources to make sense of their situations, their surroundings, and their lives. In more recent work she studies the participation of people with dementia in a variety of situations and with varying resources and needs, and especially in self-help group meetings. She applies what could perhaps be called an ethnographic social interactionist approach with a special interest in the perspectives of the persons with dementia. Together with coworkers she is currently developing a research program and an international network on citizenship and dementia.

Introduction

Beyond Loss: Dementia, Identity, Personhood

LARS-CHRISTER HYDÉN, HILDE LINDEMANN, AND JENS BROCKMEIER

Over the next decades, the number of persons diagnosed with age-related dementia worldwide will dramatically increase. For the most part, this is a consequence of demographic changes: more people are living longer. Moreover, such diagnoses are now possible at an earlier stage, which means that people with dementia will likely also live longer after diagnosis and spend a not inconsiderable part of the time at home and in their communities. Statistics show that they are mostly cared for by a spouse or adult child. The changing picture of age-related dementia gives rise to new and urgent research questions; in particular, it will be important to increase our knowledge about the way persons with dementia themselves experience and cope with the progressing disease. Dementia is not only a social phenomenon, but also a subjective experience. It is a way of life. How do affected people live that life satisfactorily? What kind of support do they themselves request so that their lives will go as well as they can? These and other questions have to be explored in order to develop more advanced, more social, and more humane forms of care. Generally, there is a need for more public knowledge about dementia as a complex subjective experience and form of life. Rather than focusing exclusively on the person diagnosed with dementia as an isolated patient, a target of care, it will become crucial to see the person as an agent of his or her own life and, hence, as an agent of care, even under what are sometimes extremely difficult conditions.

Central in this endeavor is a vision that goes beyond the individual's loss—especially the loss of cognitive and linguistic abilities—and rather sees both personhood and identity in more complex terms of transformation and change. Furthermore, it is a vision in which these processes of transformation and change typically take place in collaboration with other persons, significant others as well as care professionals. There is rarely ever a completely isolated person with dementia, although this image is widespread. Accordingly, the authors in this collection explore a number of new empirical, theoretical, and methodological perspectives that will be central to both research and clinical practice concerned with age-related dementia in the years to come. Three general areas or themes are identified as being of particular importance and interest:

1. *Persons, personhood, and dignity*: Understanding the person with dementia in a way that foregrounds his or her remaining abilities.
2. *Identity, agency, embodiment*: Viewing identity and self as part of the remaining agentive abilities of the person with dementia.
3. *Communication, family, and institutions*: Exploring modes of social interaction, be it in the family or an institution of care, that allow persons with dementia to communicate who they are through a variety of practices, including conversation, storytelling, art, and literature.

These three areas are addressed in different ways—disciplinarily, theoretically, clinically—by the authors in this volume. The papers in the first section take up the basic notions of persons, personhood, and dignity. If personhood is a form of being and a practice into which we are initiated so early in life that it becomes second nature to us, it would seem that when Alzheimer's disease (AD) or some other dementing disease strips us of our second natures, we can no longer be or participate in it. This, the philosopher Hilde Lindemann argues, would be the tragedy of AD: the disease reduces the individual to a nonperson. In her chapter, "Second Nature and the Tragedy of Alzheimer's," Lindemann claims that this line of thinking is false. After a historical examination of the concept of second nature, Lindemann argues that while second nature is not essential to personhood, so that its loss cannot deprive the individual with dementia of his or her personhood, the process by which we acquire our second natures shows us something interesting and important about the essentially social nature of persons. She concludes by offering reasons why, when those with AD have lost their second natures, we are morally responsible for "holding them in personhood."

In his chapter "The Person with Dementia as Understood through Stern's Critical Personalism," psychologist Steven R. Sabat presents William Stern's "personalistic" view of individuals as self-directed, goal-seeking agents who use their bodies as instruments with which to realize their intentions, achieve goals, and interact with the world in ways that maintain their dignity. Transcribed conversations with people diagnosed with moderate to severe AD, along with their actions in the social world, are shown to reflect a host of intact cognitive and social abilities that are articulated by Stern as being part and parcel of human life. These intact abilities are not measured by the standard neuropsychological tests of cognitive function that are used to help define the severity of cognitive decline attributable to AD. As a result, because the remaining intact cognitive and social abilities articulated by Stern are so poorly understood, people with moderate to severe AD are underestimated in terms of their ability to interact with and find meaning in their social world and in their own lives. Underestimation of such people can lead to their being treated in dysfunctional ways, further exacerbating their difficulties and compromising the efforts of care partners. Conversely, recognizing Sternian forms of cognitive abilities can lead to an enhancement of the quality of life of people diagnosed, as well as that of their care partners.

In the chapter "Dignity and Dementia," the philosopher Lennart Nordenfelt offers a comprehensive concept of dignity that addresses the condition of persons with dementia. He proposes a conceptual framework consisting of four main types of dignity: the dignity of merit, the dignity of moral stature, the dignity of identity, and the specifically human dignity of *Menschenwürde*. He tries to show how all these types of dignity are relevant for the analysis of the care of elderly persons, including persons with dementia, and concludes that a special variant of dignity of identity, the dignity of wisdom, can be attributed not only to older people in general but also to persons with dementia.

Most people with dementia are cared for within the family, often by a spouse. In the concluding paper in Part I, "'I'm his wife, not his carer!' Dignity and Couplehood in Dementia," Ingrid Hellström discusses the concept of dignity in the context of spousal relationships. The chapter is based on a longitudinal interview study with three couples living with dementia, over five years; all with different living conditions, yet all balancing their own and their spouse's actions in everyday life. An appreciation of the nature of dyadic relationships is essential to a full understanding of the way in which people adjust to dementia. Hellström argues that the relationship between the person with dementia and others, particularly family caregivers, is a key factor in maintaining a sense of self and personhood for the person, which in turn preserves the person's dignity. The spouses with dementia actively avoid situations that could have an effect on their dignity, and the cognitively intact spouses try to maintain the involvement of the ill partners and to stress former achievements.

The papers in the second section address matters of identity, agency, and embodiment. Much of the research on dementia has argued that the loss of cognitive and linguistic abilities will result in a loss of selfhood and identity. One of the typical features of AD is the loss of memory, something that has become a metonymic trope for dementia in general. The idea of memory loss is discussed by the philosopher and psychologist Jens Brockmeier in the chapter "Questions of Meaning: Memory, Dementia, and the Postautobiographical Perspective." He challenges the traditional neuropsychological and psychiatric assumption that dementia is grounded in the pathological dissolution of a specific, well-defined entity called "memory." According to this assumption, it is especially autobiographical memory that provides the basis for personal identity, mostly understood as continuity and coherence in time. This idea has been most influential in Western thought (and clinical practice), so much so that "memory disorders" as found in dementia are commonly seen as threatening a person's identity. Drawing on recent neuroscientific research on memory, Brockmeier offers a critique of this conception, including the traditional psychological and neuroscientific concept of memory as a more or less substantial biological entity that encodes, stores, and retrieves experience. He also points out what the traditional conception of autobiographical memory excludes: a view that conceives of persons, their identities, and their sense of time in an embodied and socially embedded way, a view that localizes processes of remembering and identity formation not solely in the brain but in cultural forms of life. That is, the traditional conception excludes a view of one's identity or sense of self that is grounded in practices of meaning-making. Examining some narrative examples of such practices, the chapter concludes that our gestalts of identity and autobiographical memory—both in healthy individuals and in individuals suffering from dementia—are better understood as intersubjective meaning-constructions than as biological configurations.

In her chapter "Everyday dramas: Comparing life with dementia and acquired brain injury," the neuropsychologist Maria I. Medved argues that regardless of whether an individual is suffering from neurodegeneration or neurotrauma, the cognitive changes that take place extend beyond the individual and into social domains. Most often this is the domain of one's family. Shared among the different family members is the effort to figure out what the affected person can and can no longer do; this in turn will influence both how the person sees herself and how others see her. The attempt to track the person's shifting identity is enacted in everyday life in an ongoing interpretation of what a "symptom" might be and what it might mean for various family members. There are commonalities across families, irrespective of whether the cognitive challenges are due to injury or dementia, regarding how this is accomplished. At the same time, however, there are fundamental differences between neurodegeneration and neurotrauma, as the former involves gradual cognitive decline, whereas the latter comes with the chance of recovery. Medved examines aspects of meaning-making processes in relation to identity and personhood by presenting a comparative case analysis of two families, one dealing with AD and the other with stroke.

All chapters of this book take a critical stance toward the view that cognitive abilities, selfhood, and identity are supposedly located inside the brain. It also has been challenged by a phenomenologically grounded critique to the effect that cognitive resources as well as selfhood and identity are embodied. The anthropologist Pia C. Kontos points out that the body has not been well incorporated into the discussion among diverse conceptions of the self and the experience of having AD. In the chapter "Musical Embodiment, Selfhood, and Dementia" she outlines a theory of identity that captures the ways in which selfhood is embodied and reproduced nondiscursively through our corporeal actions. This perspective takes its theoretical bearings from combining the pragmatic and epistemological primacy of cultural structures in Bourdieu's theory of practice with Merleau-Ponty's philosophy of the primordial source of agency. Although Merleau-Ponty's notion of the primordial body may seem elemental in its contribution to selfhood, Kontos argues that it not only allows us to understand the embodiment of the sociocultural sources of selfhood, but also sustains the importance of these sociocultural dispositions. Incorporating the body into a rethinking of personhood in dementia is not merely an exercise in philosophical anthropology, but one that has important implications for improving dementia care practice.

The body and embodied abilities are also the focus of Alison Phinney's chapter "As the Body Speaks: Creative Activity in Dementia." She too draws on a phenomenological perspective on personhood that emphasizes its dialogical and embodied character, but with a different accent. In order to uncover new ways of understanding dementia and its influence on people's lives, Phinney uses empirical findings from a series of four research studies conducted with people with mild to moderate dementia. These studies provide a rich body of qualitative data, including interviews and videotaped observations from seven participants who identified their involvement in creative activity as a central feature in their everyday lives. The analysis throws new light on how creative activity is experienced in and through the lived body, revealing how such experiences allow embodied meaning to persist through identity, social connection, and emotional engagement.

Early diagnosis of dementia or even prestages of dementia mostly implies that persons will live with their diagnosis in their family, thus bringing to the fore issues of family life and communication at home and in institutional contexts. The third section of the book explores these issues. Living with dementia entails developing and changing the way interaction is organized. When a family member or spouse gradually loses the ability both to tell stories and to remember shared events and stories due to AD, this is often experienced as very distressing. The social psychologist Lars-Christer Hydén argues that most spouses and family members try to remedy the communicative problems caused by progressing AD by taking over some of the functions lost by the person with AD. In his chapter "How to do Things with Others: Joint Activities Involving Persons with Alzheimer's Disease," he suggests that storytelling involving persons with AD can be seen as a "collaborative activity": two tellers contribute to the story, although one of the storytellers assumes more responsibility for both elaborating and pursuing the storyline as well as for organizing the interaction.

By scaffolding the collaboration, both participants may successfully be able to jointly tell a story. At the same time, the cognitive and linguistic troubles that are identified by both participants in the interaction pose the constant threat that the person with AD will fall out of the conversation and become a nonparticipant. A great deal of repair work is needed to help the person with AD to remain an active participant and subject of interaction.

The linguist Camilla Lindholm, in her chapter "Comprehension in Interaction: Communication at a Day-care Center," points out that questions constitute a vital area of research on communication between caregivers and elderly with dementia. In interaction with persons with AD, one should avoid open-ended questions and instead use yes-no questions or alternative questions; this is what professional guidelines suggest. However, Lindholm, in examining situations where a question posed by a caregiver fails to receive an immediate response, reports that the success or failure of a question sequence depends more on how participants work together to construct meaning than on the specific question format. Thus, to improve mutual understanding in interaction with people with dementia, caregivers need to be careful not only about the format of their question, but also about how and when to provide support to conversationalists.

In the chapter "'Familyhood' and Young-onset Dementia: Using Narrative and Biography to Understand Longitudinal Adjustment to the Diagnosis," Pamela Roach, John Keady, and Penny Bee maintain that when younger persons with dementia receive a diagnosis, they often become the sole therapeutic unit of engagement for clinical services. Consequently, artificial boundaries appear that separate them from their families, despite the repercussion of the diagnosis felt throughout the family. Keeping younger people with dementia in the family role they adopted prior to diagnosis is, however, essential if they are to move beyond the feelings of loss and helplessness that may surround the disclosure. This chapter outlines the results of an eighteen-month longitudinal study that involved five younger people with dementia and their family members, tracking postdiagnostic transitions and adjustments that allow them to maintain a sense of balance within the family. The authors discuss details of the narrative approach adopted for the study, as well as the importance of social relationships. The chapter closes with implications for future improvements in the provision of high-quality dementia care for younger people with dementia and their families.

Many persons with a dementia diagnosis live independently for a considerable time, yet little is known of how persons with early stage dementia perceive the future and cope with the evolving disease. Using positioning theory, in "The Subjectivity of Disorientation: Moral Stakes and Concerns," Linda Örulv explores nuances of the subjective experience of disorientation as expressed in social interaction in the context of dementia residential care. In this case study, the focus is on residents' personal stakes and concerns about spatiality and place as they simultaneously position themselves in relation to moral frameworks. The analysis reveals that matters of staying, leaving, returning, going somewhere, and recognizing a place raise an abundance of moral concerns that may cause much anxiety. Being on one's way somewhere, in a disoriented manner, may be an attempt to seek out an arena offering better opportunity for moral action as a morally responsible person. Seemingly confused speech may be a strategy for claiming moral agency, reflecting the need to justify and legitimize one's presence in the facility. The study suggests a care paradigm more sensitive to resident's moral concerns and stakes in daily life, taking seriously their need for meaning-driven and agentive action in line with deeply rooted personal values.

Underlying all chapters of this volume is the thesis that in order to understand the forms of life and experience of people with dementia we have to go beyond the deeply ingrained focus on the individual and on individual losses, whether these are considered in cognitive, linguistic, social, or moral terms. Instead, the goal of these papers is to view personhood and identity in a new light: as complex processes of transformation and change, processes that typically take place in close interaction and collaboration with other persons. We believe that this goal comes particularly to the fore in the three areas of research in which these chapters contribute new insights, thoughts, and suggestions: first, the understanding of persons with dementia in a way that foregrounds their remaining abilities; second, the conceptualization of identity and self as part of the remaining agentive abilities of persons with dementia; and third, the exploration of modes of social interaction, in the family and institutions of care, that allow persons with dementia to communicate who they are through a variety of practices, including conversation, storytelling, art, and literature. Viewing people with dementia through the lens of this research shows us something that people with dementia urgently need those around them to see: that they—like the rest of us—are agents of their lives, and that they—like the rest of us—need the cooperation of others to live as well and fully as possible.

Acknowledgments

Earlier versions of most of the chapters in this volume were originally presented at the workshop "Dementia, Identity, Personhood," Linköping University, Sweden, in October 2010. The Swedish Council for Working Life and Social Research and The Swedish Research Council generously supported the workshop.

Part One

PERSONS, PERSONHOOD, AND DIGNITY

1

Second Nature and the Tragedy of Alzheimer's

HILDE LINDEMANN

An insistent sound somewhere. She swam up out of a deep warm sleep and fumbled on the nightstand for the telephone. What time was it, anyway? The phone display read a little after three in the morning.

"Hello?"

"Ms. Mencken?" The voice was unfamiliar.

"Yes? Who's calling?"

"I'm Meredith Whitehall, the night supervisor at The Pines—"

Oh dear god. It was Mom.

"—and I'm afraid your mother isn't well. She's very agitated and asking for you, and we think it might help if you—"

"I'll be right there."

Kate pulled on jeans and a sweatshirt, pushed her feet into a pair of shoes, and found the car keys. This was the third time in two months that she'd received such a call, though never so late at night. She didn't mind going, really she didn't, she'd asked the staff to please let her know any time Mom needed her. As she drove down the dark highway, the guilty despair that had dogged her constantly since she'd moved her mother into the nursing home was lifted for a moment by a flicker of hope. What if Mom had asked for her by name? The old woman didn't have many words left anymore. Please let her call me Kate just one last time.

She could hear the wailing all the way down the corridor. Running to her mother's room, she flung the door open to see all the lights on, her mother wild-eyed in a corner, two aides trying to calm her, and her roommate sitting bolt upright in bed, sobbing.

Kate ran to her mom. "What's all this noise, Sweetheart?"

It was a bad move. Panicked, her mother swung a punch, hitting Kate squarely in the mouth. The wailing ascended into a shriek and then it was kicks and more punches and blood everywhere until the aides managed to restrain the frightened woman. But they couldn't restrain her tongue. She screamed abuse at Kate, using filthy epithets Kate didn't even know she knew, her face contorted with hate as she tried to lunge at her daughter again. Kate backed out of the room, the taste of blood hot in her mouth. Weeping silently, she cupped one hand under her chin and carefully spat out a tooth.

This elderly woman is not, of course, morally responsible for the vicious attack on her daughter—the amyloid plaques building up in her brain have not only eaten away most of her words, they have destroyed her moral agency. Once she was a loving mother, kind, gentle, proud of her dear Kate. Now Alzheimer's disease has destroyed most of those ways of being. As the woman's dementia grows more pronounced, the losses mount up until her very self is gone. And along with her self, she loses her second nature.

"We tend to be forgetful," remarks John McDowell, "of the very idea of second nature" (McDowell 1996, 85). It's a pity, really, as second nature is such a useful concept. Aristotle draws on it in his account of how ethical character is formed. Jean-Jacques Rousseau invokes it to solve the problem of how autonomous individuals can obey only themselves and yet unite with others to live under a rule of law. McDowell uses it to explain how rational minds connect to the natural world. In this chapter I want to use it too, along with my own riff on Sara Ruddick's concept of preservative love, to offer an account of what happens to one's status as a person when one is in the later stages of a progressive dementia. If the practice of expressing our personhood and recognizing it in others is second nature to us, it would seem that when Alzheimer's or some other dementing disease takes away our second natures, we can no longer participate in the practice; the disease could be thought to reduce the individual to a nonperson. But this conclusion is false. I'll argue that after second nature has departed, the same force that imbued us with it in the first place can keep our personhood intact. It's a species of preservative love.

Second Nature

In Aristotle's *Ethics*, virtue of character requires a properly formed intellect. Morality, on his view, involves reasons for action, and these exist independently of our awareness of them, whether or not we are responsive to them. We come to see what those reasons are by acquiring "practical wisdom" (*phronesis*)—the faculty that lets us recognize and reflect on the rational requirements of morality, and opens our eyes to the system of concepts and ways of proceeding that make the demands of morality intelligible to us.

We acquire *phronesis* by a decent upbringing, which instills good habits in us. "We must start," says Aristotle, "from what is knowable to us. Consequently, in order to listen appropriately to discussion about what is fine and just... one must have been well brought up. For the starting point is *that* it is so, and if this were sufficiently clear to us—well, in that case there will be no need to know in addition *why*. But such a person either has the relevant first principles, or might easily grasp them" (Aristotle 1941, 1095b, 4–9). This upbringing is crucial, for we are not naturally virtuous: "None of the excellences of character comes about in us by nature; for no natural way of being is changed through habituation.... The excellences develop in us neither by nature nor contrary to nature, but because we are naturally able to receive them and are brought to completion by means of habituation" (Aristotle 1941, 1103a, 20–26).

Notice that for Aristotle, ethical formation takes place within the *polis*. The well-ordered society provides the conditions under which sound moral training can take place: "But it is hard for someone to get the correct guidance towards excellence, from childhood on, if he has not been brought up under laws that aim at that effect; for a moderate and resistant way of life is not pleasant for most people, especially when they are young" (Aristotle 1941, 1179b, 31–34). Each of us, then, is dependent on the state as well as some number of others for the coaching, correcting, showing by example, and other forms of training by which we learn how to "do" morality. The habits of thought and action resulting from this training can be understood as second nature.

Rousseau too was interested in ethical formation, but he had a different problem: whereas Aristotle's difficulty was to explain how we can attain moral virtue if none of it arises in us by nature, Rousseau had to reconcile the Enlightenment insistence on self-legislation as the source of moral legitimacy with the need for social order. Dissatisfied with theories that looked to either God or nature as the ultimate ground of normativity, Enlightenment theorists sought to put morality on a secular and humanist footing. In Max Weber's fine term, Enlightenment nature became "disenchanted," emptied of the norms and values that on an Aristotelian ethics could anchor and justify moral claims. The free, autonomous individual answered to no one and nothing but himself, for only in that way could he be free. But now the authority of the nation-state over its citizens became deeply problematic. If the individual made his own laws, it was hard to see how he could subject himself to the laws of another—whether imposed by majority vote, a constitutional legislator, or a tyrant. State legislation, it seemed, could only be contingent, legitimately binding individuals only if they happened to choose the same laws for themselves. As Rousseau famously put it, "The problem is to find a form of association which will defend and protect with the whole common force the person and goods of each associate, and in which each, while uniting himself with all, may still obey himself alone, and remain as free as before" (Rousseau 1987, 24).

The solution favored by most Enlightenment philosophers was to find a way for individuals to participate jointly in a "general will" that is both the will of each and the will of all, so that there could be no conflict between self-legislation and the laws of the state. Kant, for example, theorized that transcendental Reason dictates universally binding moral norms to which, on pain of irrationality, we must freely subject ourselves. For him, the general will is reason itself, and our freedom consists in identifying ourselves with our rationality. Rousseau, however, had to take a different approach: his picture of human beings was of earth-bound, embodied, and passionate as well as rational individuals who are products of their time and place, so he couldn't look to transcendental reason to unite them. Instead, he argued that human beings' biological first natures must be remade, overlaid with socially inculcated *second* natures that incline them to choose principles of social cooperation. Because these choices are voluntary, they are free, and because they conduce to social harmony, they don't conflict with the laws of the state.

John McDowell's problem is more basic than either Aristotle's or Rousseau's. His question is not how can we be moral, nor even how can we have both freedom and social harmony, but rather, how can rational beings exist in the natural world at all. If, as the Enlightenment philosophers thought, nature is disenchanted, deprived of the meaningful relations that constitute rationality—if, that is to say, the "space of reasons," as McDowell calls it, has no connection whatever to the natural "realm of law"—then our minds can't be constrained by the world, and we have no way of justifying any of our beliefs about it. The natural realm could certainly cause us to have sensory experiences—I stub my toe on a rock, for example—but the content of our experience would be brutally natural, quite separate from the conceptual content proper to beliefs and judgments.

The "space of reasons" to which beliefs belong is constituted by "relations such as implication or probabilification" (McDowell 1996, 7). Beliefs are "spontaneous," in that we are free to rationally examine and change all the elements in our conception of the world, but they can be justified only by other beliefs. As Donald Davidson has it, "nothing can count as a reason for holding a belief except another belief" (Davidson 1986, 310). And therein lies the difficulty. If the world is completely separate from the mind, it can't give us reasons for what we believe. And if the mind is completely separate from the world, then our beliefs are unbounded, free to fly off in every direction. They "degenerate into moves in a self-contained game" (McDowell 1996, 5) or "a frictionless spinning in a void" (McDowell 1996, 11). But surely judgments of nature as we experience it must be grounded in a way that relates them to a reality outside our minds, or they can't be a source of knowledge.

Worse still, given this opposition between the space of reasons and the realm of law, it becomes impossible to see how our sensory intake of the world, which we surely share with other natural animals, can be connected to conceptual thought at all. So what we have here are two problems: the epistemological problem of how conceptual thought can be *about* sensible nature, and the ontological problem of how minds can *exist* in sensible nature. Rationality threatens, as it were, to be "extruded" from nature, with no way to bridge the gap between the two.

McDowell's solution is to reflect on Aristotle's ethics. Rather than dualistically set the space of reasons over against our animal nature, he argues, we ought to appreciate the Aristotelian insight into our *second* nature as rational animals. When we do that, we can see that initiation into the space of reasons is simply an ordinary part of becoming mature adults. Through many kinds of socialization, our natural or animal processes (such as sensory perception) become infused with conceptual meaning: we distinguish the patch of lighter and darker blues from its surroundings and see it as a shirt. This "seeing as" produces knowledge because the world actually is organized according to the concepts by which we understand it: "For a perceiver with capacities of [reason]," he writes, "the environment is...the bit of objective reality that is within her perceptual and practical reach. It is that for her because she can conceive it in ways that display it as that" (McDowell 1996, 116). On McDowell's view, then, the meaningless realm of law conceived as the object of modern natural science isn't all there is to nature. Nature also includes rational animals, whose second nature, acquired through initiation into the space of reason, gives them (us) a "foothold in the realm of law" and thereby sets welcome limits on the free interplay of ideas.

How does that initiation take place? An absolutely central element in the ordinary maturation of human beings is the acquisition of language. In learning language—spoken, written, or sign—a child learns far more than what specific words mean. Stanley Cavell puts it this way:

> When you say "I love my love" the child may learn the meaning of the word 'love' and what love is. I.e., that (*what you do*) will *be* love in the child's world, and if it is mixed with resentment and intimidation, then love is a mixture of resentment and intimidation, and when love is sought *that* will be sought. When you say "I'll take you tomorrow, I promise," the child begins to learn what temporal durations are, and what trust is, and what you do will show what trust is worth. When you say "Put on your sweater," the child learns what commands are and what *authority* is, and if giving orders is something that creates anxiety

for you, then authorities are anxious, authority itself uncertain. Of course, hopefully, the person, growing, will learn other things about these concepts and 'objects' also. They will grow gradually as the child's world grows. (Cavell 1961, 214)

Through learning language children learn the rational connections between concepts, but they also acquire the things that undergird rationality: they get a sense for what is ordinary or out of the common, what they can take for granted and what requires investigation, how "we" do things and how to tell who counts as "we." As Cavell was later to put it,

We learn and teach words in certain contexts, and then we are expected, and expect others, to be able to project them into further contexts. Nothing insures that this projection will take place (in particular, not the grasping of universals nor the grasping of a book of rules), just as nothing insures that we will make, and understand, the same projections. That on the whole we do is a matter of our sharing routes of interest and feeling, modes of response, senses of humor and of significance and of fulfillment, of what is outrageous, of what is similar to what else, what a rebuke, what forgiveness, of when an utterance is an assertion, when an appeal, when an explanation—all the whirl of organism Wittgenstein calls "forms of life." Human speech and activity, sanity and community, rest on nothing more, but nothing less, than this. It is a vision as simple as it is difficult, and as difficult as it is (and because it is) terrifying. (Cavell 1969, 52)

And *why* do we share routes of interest and feeling, modes of response, senses of humor and of significance and of fulfillment? Because the people around us teach us to do so—these things become a part of our second natures. It seems, then, that second natures give us our very selves: we are who we are because of them. Moreover, and just as fundamentally, our second natures give us the world. They make our experiences of it intelligible, and this in turn allows us to act purposefully in it, according to the reasons that are there.

The Practice of Personhood

I want to build on MacDowell's conception of second nature by connecting it to the practice of personhood. To treat someone as a person does not involve knowing that "this is a person," but rather consists in taking up a certain attitude or stance toward her. Implicit in this stance is the recognition that the person has certain rights, is properly the object of various moral duties, and so on, and to that extent, we can speak of the attitude as a moral attitude. But it's also more than that. It includes taking for granted that persons wear clothes and are given names rather than numbers, or that they are to be referred to as "who" instead of "what." The stance we take toward persons is one we learn, and we learn it so early and so thoroughly that it becomes second nature.

In the *Philosophical Investigations,* Ludwig Wittgenstein remarks that "the human body is the best picture of the human soul" (Wittgenstein 2001, 152). All of the section containing this remark deals with how we recognize and respond to people's so-called psychological or mental states—what we tend to think of as people's inner lives. It's people's bodies that express whether they are excited, puzzled, or interested; whether they are amused, fearful, or determined. So, in reading their bodies—their postures, gestures, and expressions—we are simultaneously reading what's "in" their minds. And it's our ability to read human bodies in this way that allows us to see human beings as personalities rather than as furniture, plants, or pets (Walker 1998, 181).

In explaining *how* we read bodies Wittgenstein insists that this is something we have had to learn. As Margaret Urban Walker puts it, "We have to grasp the code of recognition (what Wittgenstein called the 'method of projection' or the 'application' of a kind of picture) that connects certain displays with certain meanings, and so makes a picture show what it does" (Walker 1998, 182). What's there to be read (or misunderstood) is the changing procession of sensations, emotions, beliefs, attitudes, wishes, misgivings, and other mental states that cross a human consciousness. The capacity to generate selected items in this procession has been taken by some philosophers to be either necessary or sufficient for personhood, but I want to suggest instead that the psychological states themselves are the stuff around which personhood coalesces. If we take seriously, as I believe we must, that these states receive physical expression and are socially mediated, and that persons too are essentially social, then, rather than tying personhood solely to capabilities and competencies residing within the individual, we have to see it as largely also an interpersonal achievement.

Pushing Wittgenstein's "picture" remark one step further, I argue that our psychological states, their bodily representations, others' uptake of these representations, and the treatment based on that uptake all play a part in the formation and maintenance of personhood. Put more precisely, my claim is that personhood just *is* the bodily expression of the feelings, thoughts, desires, and intentions that constitute a human personality, as recognized by others, who then respond in certain ways to what they see. *Recognition* includes establishing a personal identity by engaging in the narrative activity that constitutes our sense of who the person is. *Response* includes the attitudes and actions we take toward the person—what we do to or for the person and what we expect from the person—on the basis of that identity-constituting, narrative activity (Nelson 2001). The bodily depiction of the succession of mental states and its uptake by others in the form of recognition and response make up what can be called the social practice of personhood, the practice on which all other social practices rest.

We begin to be initiated into this practice in infancy. Even babies recognize and respond to people's faces; so much seems to be a part of our animal natures. Building on that and other innate capacities, the adults and older children who interact with the baby give it the conceptual resources—the language—that allow it to understand what the human face expresses. As they learn to talk, beginning around eleven months of age (Briesch et al. 2008), babies make their first clumsy forays into the practice of personhood.

Of course, it takes more than language to become an adept practitioner. It may be that a capacity for empathy is required for the practice, along with other capacities that not all human beings share. My point here, however, is merely that full participation in the expressions, recognitions, and responses that constitute personhood ordinarily become second nature, as automatic and unthinking as color recognition, counting, or speech.

The Tragedy of Alzheimer's

In any progressive dementia, a point is reached when speech begins to misfire, becoming clumsy, then garbled, and finally vanishes altogether. Kate's mother loses her conceptual grip, forgetting what a key is for, or what goes in a refrigerator. She loses her sense of what is ridiculous; what is kind, cruel, or courageous; and when an utterance is an assertion, an appeal, an explanation. She can no longer read other people's bodily expressions of their feelings, desires, or intentions, and her inability to make sense of them means she can't respond to them properly. She loses her understanding of who she herself is: the tissue of stories by which she has made sense of her own life gradually or suddenly come unraveled, hanging in tatters like a moth-eaten tapestry (Gillett 2002, 27). The disease destroys her second nature, and with it, her self.

Once Kate's mother is stripped of her second nature and with it her capacity to participate in personhood, it would seem that she is condemned to the status of a nonperson, and that is to have no kind of human life at all. This, we might conclude, is the tragedy of Alzheimer's. The disease takes away everything that matters about being human.

I argue that this conclusion is false. We can see it is false if we reflect on the process whereby she gained her second nature in the first place. It took a great many people—indeed, the customs and institutions of an entire society—to give her the language, the shared interest and feeling, the modes of response, the sense of right and wrong, and all the rest of it that constituted her second nature. Which is to say, it took many others' recognition and response to teach her how to engage in personhood.

But when she was so young that she could not yet take part in the practice herself, Kate's mother was *held* in personhood by the people who cared for her. Then, her ability to express frustration, pleasure, or other mental states gave her parents and other caregivers something on which to anchor their recognition and response—they engaged in a one-sided practice of personhood. Now that she once again lacks the capacity for active participation in the practice of personhood, she may still retain enough mental functioning to be held in personhood by her loved ones or by kind and caring professionals. This holding, I maintain, is a kind of preservative love. Ruddick reserved that term for the maternal work of keeping children safe from *physical* harm (Ruddick 1989). I extend it, here, to encompass safekeeping from *moral* harm—the harm of being cast out of the special social and moral status accorded to persons. To fail to hold human beings in personhood—to treat them as nonpersons, as nothing more than a body to be washed, clothed, and fed, for example—is to cut them off from the social relationships that contribute heavily to their humanity. And to do it to someone who can still be held in personhood would be the real tragedy of Alzheimer's.

Is it a Tragedy?

It can be objected that for people with Alzheimer's who no longer have a second nature, not being held in personhood is no tragedy. To explain how this could be, let us consider a different sort of case, in which the refusal to hold in personhood someone who lacks a second nature clearly *is* a tragedy.

In Werner Herzog's 1974 film *Jeder für sich und Gott gegen alle* (in English *The Enigma of Kaspar Hauser*), which is closely based on events that actually took place in the early years of the nineteenth century, the baby Kaspar is snatched from his cradle and forced to live for the next seventeen years imprisoned in a dark cell, with no human companionship of any kind. The only person he ever sees is a man in a black overcoat and top hat, who gives him bread and water. In 1828 (although Kaspar of course has no idea what year it is, or even what a year is), the man pulls Kaspar out of his cell, teaches him to write his name, walk, and say a few phrases, and abandons him on a street in Nuremberg. The object of much curiosity, he becomes an exhibit in a circus before the kindly Herr Daumer rescues him, teaches him to read and write, and exposes him to music. Kaspar learns quickly, but he is always very strange, unfit to live on his own and requiring constant care.

Kaspar never acquired a second nature, and so never fully became a person. All he has is his animal nature, which he shares with every other beast in the wild. And as Alison Gopnik observes, "A wild animal or a wildflower is fully an animal or a flower. But a wild child, like the famous Wild Child of Aveyron, is a damaged and injured child" (Gopnik 2009, 67). The tragedy here, of course, is that he need not have been damaged. Had he not been left utterly alone all those years, he could have lived as persons do, caring for and about others, participating in civic life, practicing a trade or a profession, enjoying his evenings in a tavern, perhaps marrying and having children. In short, he could have had a *human* life. That he did not, because he was torn from those who would have held him in personhood until he was old enough to be a person on his own, was a terrible wrong.

Must we hold others in personhood? If the inability to have a life as a person is to have no kind of human life at all, and we have a right to life, it would seem we have a right to a human life. If so, then the requirement to hold in personhood shares its justification with the requirement not to murder, and is equally stringent.

It could be objected, however, along the lines of the famous Judith Jarvis Thomson argument, that even if a right to life as a person could be established, that does not yet establish your right to my services in holding you in it (Thomson 1971). All it would seem to establish is that I may not do anything—imprison you for years in a dark cell, for instance—that keeps you from holding yourself there. Most calls on people that carry imperatival force require us to *refrain* from acting, and in any case, all rights have boundaries: the right to swing my fist, as they say, ends at your nose.

One problem with the Thomson-style objection is that there are plenty of positive calls on us that are moral requirements, ranging all the way from the obligation to rescue the toddler drowning in the shallow pond, to the duty to keep your promises. The better reason to see holding in personhood as obligatory, however, is that a human life, to borrow Michael Bratman's lovely phrase, is a shared cooperative activity, characterized by mutual responsiveness, commitment to the joint activity, and—this is the crucial bit—commitment to mutual support (Bratman 1992, 328). If we are playing basketball, to use one of Bratman's examples, and you are on the team, then the rest of us players have to pass the ball to you, set picks for you, and do all the other things teammates are supposed to do during the game. By the same argument, if your life as a human being depends on your entering the practice of personhood and you have a right to life as a human being, then the rest of us in the practice have to commit to keeping you playing with us. After all, holding someone like Kaspar in personhood needn't take much effort: unless you stand in a special relationship to the person (for example, you are his mother), eye contact, a smile, or a nod of recognition might be all that is required. Because the stakes for that person can be so huge and the claim on you is so small, it seems as if there is indeed an obligation to engage in this kind of holding.

By contrast to people like Kaspar Hauser, however, people in the more advanced stages of Alzheimer's can never again have the experiences of personhood. Their minds have been damaged not by human agency but by the ravages of the disease, and to date there is no known repair. And so, our objector goes on to argue, as the goods of personhood are closed to them no matter what we do, it's no tragedy for them to be treated like any other damaged animal. In any case, the objector adds, they won't know the difference. For both those reasons, they haven't been wronged.

Let's start with the second reason: they won't know the difference. The assumption here is that what you don't know can't hurt you, but that strikes me as dubious. There are certainly cases in which it might be true—for example, your grown son narrowly avoided a head-on car crash the other day and didn't see any point in alarming you—but in other cases you can be wronged even if you never find out. Consider the rich aunt who died and left you half her estate, but due to the machinations of your evil cousin, who was also her lawyer, the will was suppressed and all the money went to him. You had no expectations in the matter and are delighted by his good fortune, but it seems clear that he wronged you even though you will never know it.

The trouble with the rich aunt example, however, is that while it shows that there is such a thing as an unexperienced wrong, it doesn't fit the present case. The wrong done to you in stealing your inheritance is that your interests are set back, whereas people in advanced stages of Alzheimer's don't have comparable interests. So consider a closer example: a good friend and colleague is jealous of your recent professional success. Rather than discuss it with you, she behaves toward you as she always has but behind your back she speaks contemptuously of your work to other colleagues. They aren't influenced by her slander and don't want to hurt your feelings, so they never tell you, but it seems to me that even if you never learn of her disrespectful behavior, she has wronged you all the same. Here the wrong is not that your interests have been set back—your false friend hasn't hurt your career. The harm is, rather, a respect harm. She has failed to treat you with the kindness she owes you.

At this point, the objector might reply that the wrong done in both these cases is to deprive you of any recourse. If you knew about what had been done to you, you could take certain steps: sue to regain your inheritance, for example, or break off relations with your perfidious friend. People in the late stages of Alzheimer's, by contrast, can't know or care how they are treated, so they haven't been similarly wronged. But this argument won't do. It puts the cart before the horse, because the reason you need recourse in the first place is that you *have* been wronged. To be sure, depriving you of recourse compounds the initial wrong, but that exists regardless of whether you are in a position to redress it.

That people like Kate's mother can't know or care whether they are held in personhood is a recapitulation of the first reason for denying that there is a tragedy here, namely, that the goods of personhood are closed to them. To this I want to reply that even if they are, it matters to us now how we will be treated later. Who I am *then* isn't just an old woman lying in a nursing home bed, for I am always, until I die, the being who has lived the whole of my life. To have lived it as a person is to have set a moral course for myself, expressing who I am through my actions. In that way I take, as Kant might put it, my rightful place among other citizens in the kingdom of ends. If, at the end of my life, I can no longer actively participate in the complicated practice that makes persons of us all, I would hope to be treated with the respect that is due to any citizen of that kingdom, by being held inside it.

A final thought. It isn't good for any of us to refuse to hold in personhood those who still have some capacity, however feeble, to give bodily expression to their mental states. Such refusals all too easily lead to morally suspect patterns of belief about who gets to count as a person. At some point in our existence we all lack a second nature and depend for our lives on the preservative love of those who hold us in personhood. As human history is littered with people whose neglect, abuse, and outright killing are justified on the grounds that they are nonpersons, it is better for us never to forget that we all—young and old, helpless and self-sufficient—share in the human condition, where we need all the holding we can get.

Acknowledgments

My thanks to Jamie Nelson, whose comments and criticism have, as usual, proved invaluable, and to Jens Brockmeier, whose insightful reading has made this a better chapter.

References

Aristotle. 1941. *The Basic Works of Aristotle*. Ed. Richard McKeon. New York: Random House.
Bratman, Michael. 1992. "Shared Cooperative Activity." *Philosophical Review* 101 (2): 327–341.
Briesch, Jacqueline M., Jennifer A. Schwade, and Michael H. Goldstein. 2008. "Responses to Prelinguistic Object-Directed Vocalizations Facilitate Word Learning in 1-Month-Olds."

Poster presented at the Biennial International Conference in Infant Studies, Vancouver, Canada.
Cavell, Stanley. "The Claim to Rationality." Unpublished dissertation, Harvard University, 1961.
———. 1969. *Must We Mean What We Say?* New York: Scribner.
Davidson, Donald. 1986. "A Coherence Theory of Truth and Knowledge." In *Truth and Interpretation: Perspectives on the Philosophy of Donald Davidson*. Oxford: Basil Blackwell.
Gillett, Grant. 2002. "You Always Were a Bastard." *Hastings Center Report* 32 (6): 23–28.
Gopnik, Alison. 2009. *The Philosophical Baby: What Children's Minds Tell Us About Truth, Love, and the Meaning of Life*. New York: Farrar, Straus, & Giroux.
McDowell, John. 1996. *Mind and World*. Cambridge: Harvard University Press.
Nelson, Hilde Lindemann. 2001. *Damaged Identities, Narrative Repair*. Ithaca, NY: Cornell University Press.
Rousseau, Jean-Jacques. [1762] 1987. *On the Social Contract*. Translated by D. A. Cress. Indianapolis: Hackett.
Ruddick, Sara. 1989. *Maternal Thinking: Toward a Politics of Peace*. Boston: Beacon.
Thomson, Judith Jarvis. 1971. "A Defense of Abortion." *Philosophy & Public Affairs* 1 (1): 47–66.
Walker, Margaret Urban. 1998. *Moral Understandings*. New York: Routledge.
Wittgenstein, Ludwig. [1958] 2001. *Philosophical Investigations*. Translated by G. E. M. Anscombe. 3rd ed. Malden, MA: Blackwell.

2

The Person with Dementia as Understood through Stern's Critical Personalism

STEVEN R. SABAT

The incidence of dementia is projected to grow tremendously in the coming decades. In 2007, for instance, 13% of people age seventy-one or older in the United States, roughly 3.4 million men and women, had been diagnosed with dementia, 9.7% of which was specifically of the Alzheimer's type (Plassman et al. 2007). In the absence of a cure or preventive measures, it is expected that by 2025 the percentage of people with Alzheimer's disease (AD) will increase by 30% to roughly 5.2 million people (Hebert et al. 2003). As a result, it is possible that an unnecessary and misguided use of pharmaceutical intervention, rather than the nonpharmaceutical intervention of facilitating social relationships, will have profound psychosocial and emotional effects not only on the individuals directly involved, but on the larger society including formal and informal caregivers, as well as Medicare (in the United States) and such state systems as the National Health Service in the United Kingdom. For example, people diagnosed with dementia exhibit depression and/or agitation and these are often treated with pharmaceuticals. At the same time, decades-old research (Langer and Rodin 1976) has shown that social environment can have profound effects on the cognitive and physical well-being of people living in long-term care institutions. That is to say, the quality of life of people, whether or not they have been diagnosed with dementia, involves an interaction between the person and the environment in which he or she lives.

Given this notion of recognizing the importance of an interaction between the person and the environment, in recent years we have witnessed the development of a bio-psycho-social model of dementia as a viable alternative to the biomedical model that was dominant for most of the twentieth century. The biomedical approach focuses principally on what people cannot do and explains dysfunction of all kinds as outcomes of the disease process alone, while ignoring for the most part the existence and significance of intact cognitive and social abilities displayed outside the clinical testing situation, as well as the socially dysfunctional situations experienced by the diagnosed person and the possible negative effects thereof. The bio-psycho-social model was developed in order to focus more closely on the person in terms of his or her intact selfhood; the nature and quality of his or her subjective experience; and the ways in which social situations could affect, for better as well as for worse, the person's cognitive and social abilities.[1]

It is in the interests of family and professional caregivers, as well as those of the larger society as a whole, to maximize the quality of life of people with dementia and to sustain their ability to function independently in as many ways as possible for as long as possible. In order to achieve this important goal, it is necessary to understand the subjective experience of a person diagnosed with dementia. Understanding his or her subjective experience requires that we understand the person in his or her totality, so as to be able to contextualize his or her actions and thereby comprehend the meaning of those actions. That is to say, although it is important to know *that* someone acted in this or that way, it is even more important to know *why* the person acted as he or she did. For example, a woman being given a neuropsychological test was asked to write a sentence about anything she chose—whatever came to her mind. Having determined that the test administrator was a "doctor" (it was the present author, in fact), she wrote, "It is good to hear the doctor" (Sabat 2001). During a clinical conference about her, one of the physicians opined that her sentence included a paraphasia, an unintended word or speech sound, because she said, "hear" when she actually meant, "see." After all, when we are in the immediate company of another person, we often say, "It is good to see you" as opposed to when we are chatting with someone by telephone, when we commonly say, "It's good to hear your voice." Given that the woman had been diagnosed with AD, the physician interpreted her use of the word "hear" as an instance of pathology caused by the disease.

Further investigation of the larger context of the woman's life provided reason to doubt this interpretation. In an interview, her adult daughter and primary caregiver indicated that her mother, widowed in recent years, was married for decades to a man who verbally abused her regularly. It seemed to me, that this woman who was treated in a verbally abusive way by her husband of more than forty years, might be especially sensitive to the way in which others addressed her. During the testing situation, she and I enjoyed a very warm exchange of pleasantries throughout, contrasting mightily with the way in which her husband had addressed her during their marriage. Given all this, her sentence, "It is good to hear the doctor" made perfect sense and was clearly, from her point of view, a reality that she valued. Thus we see how what a person says or does can be misinterpreted rather easily as an instance of pathology when we are not aware of the larger context of the person's life, who that person is and has been and what that person has valued and experienced. Clearly, the typical testing situation in the clinic rarely, if ever, uncovers information about the person's life story beyond what is relatively superficial demographic information.

Standard neuropsychological tests, as a result, provide only a glimpse of a very limited sample of a person's cognitive abilities. The tests often involve items of information taken out of the larger social situations of everyday life, but presented in a clinical testing situation which, for many people, can be anxiety provoking. It is commonly known that anxiety can result in a diminution of performance. Fortunately, there are still other tools with which we can begin to understand what a person says and does and why he or she may do so. These tools, which tap aspects of psychological experience beyond what can be gleaned from standard neuropsychological tests, include those provided by William Stern's Critical Personalism.

Critical Personalism

Although he was not addressing the use of neuropsychological tests in particular, Stern was very clear about the sort of limited understanding that testing can provide:

> In the first place, tests provide only a momentary snapshot of the performance capabilities of the examinee. To be sure, we seek to use the most diagnostic tests available. But even then, it will never be possible to eliminate completely the factors which can exert a momentary influence on performance (bodily indisposition, temporary lapse in attentiveness, test anxiety). Consequently, the results of the tests do not provide a sure indicator of enduring psychological characteristics of the examinee.... By their very nature, tests require the examinee to react, and for this reason can tap only reactive behaviors. Such spontaneity as might be manifested by the examinee's interests and inclinations, or in play or artistic activities or through aesthetic or ethical or religious modes of experience, escapes tests entirely and can be captured only, if at all, by the observations of sensitive persons who have spent some extended period of time with the person whose psychological profile is being constructed.... Tests yield a number on the basis of which that examinee can be located somewhere along a quantitative scale, but which obscures things qualitatively peculiar to that individual. For all of

these reasons, the methods of direct observation must always be used to supplement the test methods, and the former must be developed and refined with the same care as the latter. (Stern 1921, 3–4).

In 1929, Stern went even further: "A human being is not a mosaic and therefore cannot be described as a mosaic. All attempts to represent a person simply in terms of a sequence of test scores are fundamentally false" (Stern 1929, 63–64). Ironically, the results of neuropsychological test batteries are precisely what are used to characterize persons' abilities to think and express themselves and are used as outcome measures in drug efficacy studies.

Therefore, Stern proposed that the approach of Critical Personalism be used as a supplement to the psychometric, quantitative approach, so as to understand the person as a unified whole. In order to arrive at such an understanding, it is necessary to explore persons' interactions with the world at large, the psychological dimensions of their lives that exert powerful influences on their social interactions. The way to accomplish this, according to Stern, was through detailed case studies of individuals first and later, perhaps, to uncover from the individual level the possibility of generalities. Among the concepts that Stern advanced in his Critical Personalism was that of "Person-World and Mental-Physical Relations" and it is this concept that I shall address first.

PERSON-WORLD AND MENTAL-PHYSICAL RELATIONS

Stern believed that "the person makes use of his body as an implement in the service of his experience" (1938, 85). Thus, there was an intimate connection between the person who has goals and intentions, and the vehicle of the body, through which the person can carry out those intentions and achieve those goals. The body is also the vehicle through which the person's experience of the world becomes intelligible. Thus, from Stern's point of view, it is logical that if the brain were injured, the person's ability to act on the world to achieve goals and manifest intentions would be compromised, as would be the person's experience of the world. This would not mean that the existence of goals and intentions would be erased necessarily, but it does mean that the *ways in which* the person goes about achieving those goals may be altered. Likewise, the person's experience may be altered somewhat, but such alterations require understanding before we draw conclusions as to their meaning. The case of Dr. B is illustrative.

Dr. B was a retired professor, a scientist, diagnosed with AD four years before my association with him began. At the time of our association he was diagnosed as being in the moderate to severe stage of the illness, and he attended an adult day center two to three days per week. I explained to him that I needed his help in understanding what AD is like and he was a willing partner in this research effort. He commented that "Alzheimer's gives me fragments" and "I absorb in globs." Here, he is noting that his ability to maintain fixed, vigilant, constant attention on his surroundings has become compromised, so that he apprehends only pieces of what's transpiring. He was becoming less and less able to filter out what we would call background noise so as to focus on what was important. For instance, on one occasion he and I were sitting and talking in the staff office and at that time, there were many people coming into and going out of the office, telephones were ringing, some staff members were talking on the telephones or to one another. Finally, Dr. B shook his head out of frustration and asked if we could go elsewhere because "There are too many stimuli in here." In healthier days he, like most of us, could have sat in the office and filtered out, or inhibited his awareness of, everything other than the conversation he was having with me, but now that was not possible for him, despite the fact that he desperately wanted to do so. Thus, his body was not serving him in achieving his goal of focusing his attention. Many months later, the disease had progressed and in the same situation, he simply shut his eyes, covered his ears with his hands, and began to weep.

Without an understanding of his experience, gained over the course of many months, one could say that his weeping was an example of his being "emotionally labile" because, after all, no one said anything or did anything to him that any reasonable person would view as an inspiration for him to weep. On the other hand, if we do have an understanding of his experience, we recognize that his crying was an entirely appropriate reaction to his frustration at not being able to focus his attention as he always did in decades of adult life. Dr. B *wanted* to filter out extraneous sounds and sights, but could not achieve this goal in the usual and customary manner because the "instrument" of his body, more specifically some critical brain system, or systems, was damaged. So he resorted to other means, such as leaving the room or shutting his eyes and covering his ears, to achieve that goal. What is of great importance here is that despite AD, (a) Dr. B's intentions were coherent and intact; (b) he formulated clear goals and plans for carrying out those goals, but (c) was unable to execute those intentions as he had done during healthy days, and (d) reacted appropriately to the frustration he felt, thereby showing (e) that his actions were driven by what the situation meant to him and not by the pathology of AD. Persons whose actions are meaning-driven have been referred to as "semiotic subjects" by Shweder and Sullivan (1989). In a sense, AD was an indirect cause of his actions, but there was nothing pathological about his intentions, his goals, his ability to carry them out, or his reaction to the effects of AD.

These last points are especially important, because on the surface, Dr. B's behavior could easily appear abnormal or difficult to comprehend. Normal observers, aware of his diagnosis but not of Dr. B in his totality and not aware of the nature of his experience and its meaning to him, will tend to interpret those abnormalities as instances of pathology, seeing Dr. B as defective. Taking Stern's admonitions seriously, however, we can look beneath the surface and recognize that Dr. B's actions were not dysfunctional at all, but were logical adaptations to the situation he confronted.

In terms of "Person-World Relations," Stern notes that a person does not react in a reflexive, mechanical way to the environment, but is, instead, an active agent: "The person seeks in the world that which he *lacks*, and reacts against the world with the force of *counteraction*, whenever his own being must be asserted in opposition to the process of assimilation" (1938, 91). Although he greeted participants at the day center warmly and graciously, Dr. B refused to take part in any of the activities that were being led by staff members. He rarely engaged in conversation with other participants, preferring instead to talk with staff members or me. He could have been characterized easily as "aloof" or "uncooperative" as a result of these actions that, themselves, could be seen as being driven by the disease process. From Stern's point of view, however, a very different picture emerges. Dr. B, an academic person throughout his adult life, found the games and activities to be, as he described them, "filler." When I asked him what "filler" was, he said, "Something that doesn't mean anything." Given that he found the games and activities meaningless, almost demeaning, he refused to be part of the group, refused to be *assimilated* into the group of "day center participants," and reacted with *counteraction* to preserve his sense of self as an academic, intellectual person. He was hardly being uncooperative or aloof. He was being very much himself, the same person who never engaged in such activities in his adult life.

PERSONAL DIMENSIONS

One such dimension that Stern discusses is what he referred to as "the personal present." What we call the present time is, according to Stern, "spatio-temporally neutral; it is the unseparated here-now" and that what is here and now is always determined "according to the personal perspective" (1938, 93). What this means is that it is possible for any of us to bring into the present moment any aspect of our lives, even though one or another aspect may have been lived in what we would call "the distant past" or even the "future" in linear time. Therefore, at the present moment, a person might be diagnosed with AD, but the same person's "personal present" might include being an attorney, author, homemaker, mother, father, and so on, even though the person is not living out those aspects of life at the present time. Thus, we understand the following exchange between

Mr. K, a day center participant and the director of the day center, who was introducing Mr. K to a third person:

Mr. G (the director, to the third party): This is Mr. K. Mr. K was a lawyer.
Mr. K (interrupting): I *am* a lawyer!

It was true that although Mr. K was not a practicing attorney at this point, an extremely important part of his personal present was the fact that the dispositions of mind, education, and attitudes that were part and parcel of his being an attorney were still quite alive within him even though he had been diagnosed with AD and was attending a day center three days per week. No one had disbarred him, he was still a graduate of law school, and these characteristics were so important to him that he literally demanded that they be acknowledged. He was not "in denial" about his being part of the day center community, or "delusional" and "still thinking he's an attorney" because of AD, as he might have been characterized from a purely biomedical point of view. Rather, if we appreciate his experience of the personal present from Stern's point of view, then we appreciate that, as Stern would say, he "seeks in the world that which he lacks"—the recognition by others of who he is, in a much larger sense of the word. He was also displaying the force of "counteraction" to the process of being assimilated into a category of "once was, but no longer is, an attorney, but is now merely a day center participant with AD." To react this way is also exemplary of being a semiotic subject, because Mr. K evaluated the meaning of the situation, recognized what he wanted and needed, but lacked, in that situation, and took action to secure that which he desired. His actions, therefore, were driven by the meaning of the situation for him.

GOALS

What Dr. B and Mr. K did involved goal-directed actions. Stern viewed persons as goal-seeking agents and discussed two types of goals, the *autotelic* type and *heterotelic* type. Autotelic goals are related to the development and maintenance of the individual's selfhood, skills, and beliefs. Other goals extend beyond the individual and reach into the areas of community, family, truth, and morality. From Stern's point of view, it is impossible to understand a person's psychological experience without relating that experience to these different types of goals and their realization. When a man with severe AD said to me as I was about to administer a neuropsychological test, "Doc, ya gotta find a way to give us purpose again," he was making it very clear that the lack of purpose or goals was profoundly saddening to him. We note, therefore, that this person's cognitive ability as measured by standard tests, could not predict or elucidate the fact that he was able to think in a way that is essentially the same way that most otherwise healthy people think, for no one enjoys feeling purposeless. Kitwood (1997) referred to healthy abilities displayed by people with dementia as "indicators of relative well being," or examples of common ground between those diagnosed and those deemed to be healthy. Therefore, we need means beyond the realm of quantitative measures (standard tests) to understand the experience of people diagnosed with AD. This notion is supported quite clearly in the case of Dr. M, who was a retired academic and diagnosed with AD in the moderate to severe stage at the time of our two-year-long association. In the following conversational extract, we see her seeking an autotelic goal, one of self-development or self-maintenance in relation to her not wanting to attend support group meetings:

Dr. M: Ya! And I don't want to do that. I, I guess I don't want to go—that I don't get enough.
SRS: Oh—you don't get enough out of the group?
Dr. M: I think I don't get the group and it's not that I don't want to be in a group like that, it's that I—That's what makes me feel bad, I think. It doesn't give me anything. I don't want to go with people who...
SRS: So you're going to sit around for an hour saying, "Gee, I don't know what we're going to do, where we should go..." (this said in a tone implying the quandary she described previously in the conversation as characterizing the group sessions).
Dr. M: Yep, exactly. That is it. At least it's a part of it.
SRS: You're impatient.
Dr. M: I don't get enough. Whew! That, that uh, clarifies a lot!

Here we see Dr. M, evaluating the meaning of attending the support group, and finding it lacking in direction and purpose. She was not "getting enough" to justify going—enough meaning help, information, refreshing experience, all of which could add to her life. She had, as a result of the progress of AD, sustained many losses including her cherished ability to speak with great fluency and grace. Her word-finding problems were anathema to her and diminished her self-worth to a great degree. Thus, she sought ways to find new joys and meaning in her life—she had autotelic goals, and she reacted with "counteraction" to any attempt to include her in a stereotypic group that was defined by illness, thereby emphasizing what she lacked to her great dismay.

At the same time, Dr. M had heterotelic goals that can be seen in the following conversational extracts. During the course of our association, Dr. M indicated concern that our relationship was not reciprocal. That is, I was helping her such that she was able to express herself more fluently and was helping her to realize some autotelic goals as a result. She expressed her appreciation for that frequently, but did not want to be on the receiving end exclusively as we see in the following:

> Dr. M: Now—then, I want to tell you something, uh, that has some—I hope you're getting something out of this.
> SRS: Oh, yes! Oh yes! No question about it.
> Dr. M: Because I, I feel, I don't want to, to use your time.
> SRS: I appreciate your concern very much, but I want to assure you that this time is so important to me and you teach me so much.

Thus, one of her heterotelic goals was that she wanted to be giving something to me in our association. She was, therefore, evaluating the situation in terms of fairness and principle, and needed to know that she was giving as well as receiving and not "using" my time.

On another occasion, she encouraged me to attend one of her support group meetings, which I then did. She thought, apparently, that I could do something good for the group (a heterotelic goal) and that she would benefit also (autotelic goal). As well, she thought that my being involved with the support group would help me in my own research efforts. All of this can be seen in the following conversation in which she began by talking about her reaction to and reflections about my having come to the support group meeting. She is referring at first to my interaction with her during the support group meeting.

> Dr. M: When he, uh, when you asked me very in, in very nice, uh, knowing, knowingly, knowingly, you were a knowingly, I, I think that uh, was I—I didn't know anything in the whole wide world to do. That and then, uh, somehow it worked itself out uh, and uh, and to have seen me talk to a group and a group whom I, I don't really know as friends or, I just wanted you to know that.
> SRS: Oh, so that was good?
> Dr. M: Oh, it was *real* good.
> SRS: I'm *so* glad. I think that everybody has something, everybody has something to offer.
> Dr. M: Oh, that's very good, kid!
> SRS: To me the angels speak sometimes. You know how it is when you have that feeling that somebody's tapping you on the shoulder and saying, "Hey—would you just wake up and look at this for a minute, will ya!"
> Dr. M: (hearty laughter)

SRS: That's how I felt when the group leader asked me if I would come back. Inside my head I was saying, "Would I? Are you kidding? I would love to!"

Dr. M: I knew that! I knew that it gives you just what you're looking for. So uh, and I think it gives, gives the group some. You repeated, I mean I repeated what you had said in a sense.

SRS: Yes indeed! I think we learn more about what people *can* do (when we observe them) in rich social settings.

Dr. M: Um hum, and you can have that for the next uh…paper.

SRS: That's right!

So Dr. M has achieved a heterotelic goal by getting me involved in her support group because that would give me "just what you're looking for," help the group as well as the professional audience through my writing a journal article—my "next…paper." She made my cause her own and that, in turn, would redound to the benefit of the group, herself, and professionals as well. In this process, she was becoming something of an academic "midwife" and that proved to enhance her sense of self-worth via the realization of an autotelic and a heterotelic goal. There was nothing in her neuropsychological test profile that would have predicted anything about her ability to think and plan and act in the world to the benefit of herself and of others. At the same time, however, through the application of Stern's ideas, we see very clearly a tremendously striking dissociation between her "profile" in quantitative, standard test terms and who she is as a person in qualitative, "critical personalistic" terms in Stern's conceptual scheme.

She was even more directive, acting as something of an academic mentor, when we discussed the idea of how people can facilitate one another when they have word-finding problems. The subject began with Dr. M recounting what happened at the previous support group meeting when I addressed another member of the group in a way that helped him to respond:

Dr. M: But when you brought out that, uh, that, nobody has asked him for ages what he did.

SRS: Um hum, and then I did.

Dr. M: and I told you that earlier on he could say just a little. Now he has lost, but now he's got it back and that was so good.

SRS: If other people can learn how to help the person use the words he or she has available, if other people can learn how to listen and how to translate, then you don't have to be that quiet (in the group).

Dr. M: Um. That's nice! That's nice of you!

SRS: My goodness! We're people aren't we? Everybody, we all have our problems don't we? And we, we need each other. Nobody can do it by him or herself.
Dr. M: I would think that you would hold this part of the work that we're doing now
SRS: Um hum,
Dr. M: uh, for if you were writing the thing.
SRS: You want me to include what I just said
Dr. M: Yes, um hum
SRS: in what I'm writing.
Dr. M: Um hum.

Stern captured this situation beautifully when he wrote,

> Perhaps the last and highest secret of the human personality, [is] that it takes up the heterotelic into the autotelic. The outer goal indeed remains, after as before, directed to the not-I, but is appropriated with and formed according to one's own self. (1917, 47)

In other words, as Stern also wrote, "People must, therefore, incorporate the ends of others into their self ends" (1923, 63). Doing good for others is a way of doing good for oneself and Dr. M was clearly capable of this high order of thinking and acting despite being in the moderate to severe stage of AD.

Even though I make no attempt to generalize from the cases herein, it should be clear from the foregoing that applying Stern's personalistic ideas to the discourse of at least some people with dementia allows us to appreciate a host of intact psychological, emotional, and cognitive abilities that would be unnoticed if we were to restrict our understanding of such people to their performance on standard neuropsychological tests. We recognize, in the process, that quantitative analysis via standard tests provides us with a very limited understanding of what it means to be diagnosed with dementia. Simultaneously, we recognize that there is a very important contribution to be made by qualitative analysis. By using both approaches, we may be able to understand the person with dementia in ways that will allow us to improve that person's quality of life through nonpharmacological means. Such means are psychosocial in nature and they include helping to support the person's sense of self-worth by recognizing the person's enduring need for purpose and maintenance of dignity and self-respect, by being sensitive to the fact that the ways in which persons with dementia go about trying to achieve autotelic and heterotelic goals may be different from their approaches in healthier days, they still are working to realize such goals.

Finally, the application of Stern's personalistic approach can help formal as well as informal caregivers to avoid underestimating the cognitive and social abilities of people with dementia. This alone could lead to a diminution of what Kitwood (1997) called, "malignant social psychology," which is how Kitwood referred to the unwitting negative forms of treatment given to people with dementia such that those diagnosed are depersonalized and experience assaults on their self-worth. Such treatment often leads to depression and, in some cases, aggression, which ironically are then treated with drugs because the depression or aggression are interpreted as being caused by the disease the person has, rather than the person's reaction to the dysfunctional ways in which he or she has been treated. Understanding the fact that the person with dementia can still be a semiotic subject who has autotelic and heterotelic goals and the need to realize them can change the culture of care we provide for people with dementia in ways that help such people retain their sense of self and self-worth for longer and longer periods of time and thereby enhance their quality of life. In doing so, those of us deemed healthy who provide such care can, as a result, enhance our own feelings of self-worth and realize our own autotelic and heterotelic goals and enhance our own quality of life.

Note

1. See Kitwood 1990, 1993, 1997, 1998; Kitwood and Bredin 1992; Lyman 1989; Cotrell and Schultz 1993; Downs 1997, 2000; Bender and Cheston 1997; Harris 2002, 2012; Holst and Hallberg 2003; Sabat, 1991, 1994, 2001, 2003, 2008, 2012; Sabat and Harré 1992, 1994; Sabat and Collins 1999; Sabat and Gladstone 2010; Sabat et al. 1999; Sabat, Napolitano, and Fath 2004; Sabat and Lee 2012; Clare 2002, 2003, 2004; Kontos 2004, 2005, 2012; Hughes 2001, 2006, 2011; Hughes, Louw, and Sabat 2006; Downs and Bowers 2008; de Medeiros, Saunders, and Sabat 2012; de Medeiros et al. 2012; Campo and Chaudhury 2012; Ward et al. 2012; Doyle, de Medeiros, and Saunders 2012.

References

Bender, M. P., and R. Cheston. 1997. "Inhabitants of a Lost Kingdom: A Model of the Subjective Experiences of Dementia." *Ageing and Society* 17: 513–532.

Campo, M., and H. Chaudhury. 2012. "Informal Social Interaction Among Residents with Dementia in Special Care Units: Exploring the Role of the Physical and Social Environments." *Dementia: The International Journal of Social Research and Practice* 11: 401–423.

Clare, L. 2002. "Developing Awareness about Awareness in Early Stage Dementia." *Dementia: The International Journal of Social Research and Practice* 1: 295–312.

Clare, L. 2003. "Managing Threats to Self: Awareness in Early-Stage Alzheimer's Disease." *Social Science and Medicine* 57: 1017–1029.

Claire, L. 2004. "Awareness in Early-Stage Alzheimer's Disease: A Review of Methods and Evidence." *British Journal of Clinical Psychology* 43: 177–196.

Cotrell, V., and R. Schulz. 1993. "The Perspective of the Patient with Alzheimer's Disease: A Neglected Dimension of Dementia Research." *The Gerontologist* 33: 205–211.

de Medeiros, K., P. Saunders, P. J. Doyle, A. Mosby, and K. Van Haitsma. 2012. "Friendships among People with Dementia in Long-Term Care." *Dementia: The International Journal of Social Research and Practice* 11: 363–381.

de Medeiros, K., P. A. Saunders, and S. R. Sabat. 2012. "Friendships among People with Dementia in Long Term Care." *Dementia: The International Journal of Social Research and Practice* 11: 1–18.

Downs, M. 1997. "The Emergence of the Person in Dementia Research." *Ageing and Society* 17: 597–607.

Downs, M. 2000. "Dementia in a Socio-cultural Context: An Idea Whose Time Has Come." *Ageing and Society* 20: 369–375.

Downs, M., and B. Bowers, editors. 2008. *Excellence in Dementia Care: Research into Practice*. Open University Press/McGraw Hill: New York.

Doyle, P. J., K. de Medeiros, and P. Saunders. 2012. "Nested Social Groups within the Social Environment of Dementia Care Assisted Living Setting." *Dementia: The International Journal of Social Research and Practice* 11: 383–399.

Harris, P. B., editor. 2002. *The Person with Alzheimer's Disease: Pathways to Understanding the Experience*. Baltimore: The Johns Hopkins University Press.

Harris, P. B. 2012. "Maintaining Friendships in Early Stage Dementia: Factors to Consider." *Dementia: The International Journal of Social Research and Practice* 11: 305–314.

Hebert, L. E., Scherr, P. A., Bienias, J. L., Bennett, D. A., and Evans, D. A. 2003. "Alzheimer's Disease in the U.S. Population: Prevalence Estimates Using the 2000 Census." *Archives of Neurology*, 60: 1119–1122.

Holst, G., and I. Hallberg. 2003. "Exploring the Meaning of Everyday Life, for those suffering from Dementia." *American Journal of Alzheimer's Disease and Other Dementias* 18: 359–365.

Hughes, J. C. 2001. "Views of the Person with Dementia." *Journal of Medical Ethics* 27: 86–91.

Hughes, J. C., editor. 2006. *Palliative Care in Severe Dementia*. London: Quay Books.

Hughes, J. C. 2011. *Thinking Through Dementia*. Oxford: Oxford University Press.

Hughes, J. C., S. J. Louw, and S. R. Sabat, editors. 2006. *Dementia: Mind, Meaning, and the Person*. Oxford: Oxford University Press.

Kitwood, T. 1990. "The Dialectice of Dementia: With Particular Reference To Alzheimer's Disease." *Ageing and Society* 10 (2): 177–196.

Kitwood, T. 1993. "Towards a Theory of Dementia Care: The Interpersonal Process." *Ageing and Society* 13: 51–67.

Kitwood, T. 1997. *Dementia Reconsidered: The Person Comes First*. Buckingham: Open University Press.

Kitwood, T. 1998. "Toward a Theory of Dementia Care: Ethics And Interaction." *Journal of Clinical Ethics* 9 (1): 23–34.

Kitwood, T., and K. Bredin. 1992. "Towards a Theory of Dementia Care: Personhood and Well-Being." *Ageing and Society* 12 (1): 269–287.

Kontos, P. C. 2004. "Ethnographic Reflections on Selfhood, Embodiment, and Alzheimer's Disease." *Ageing and Society* 24 (6): 829–849.

Kontos, P. C. 2005. "Embodied Selfhood in Alzheimer's Disease: Rethinking Person-Centered Care." *Dementia: The International Journal of Social Research and Practice* 4 (4): 553–570.

Kontos, P. C. 2012. "Rethinking Sociability in Long-Term Care: An Embodied Dimension of Selfhood." *Dementia: The International Journal of Social Research and Practice* 11: 329–346.

Langer, E. J., and J. Rodin. 1976. "The Effects of Choice and Enhanced Personal Responsibility for the Aged: A Field Experiment in an Institutional Setting." *Journal of Personality and Social Psychology* 34: 191–198.

Lyman, K. 1989. "Bringing the Social Back in: A Critique of the Biomedicalization of Dementia." *Gerontologist* 29: 597–604.

Plassman, B. L., K. M. K. Langa, G. G. Fisher, S. G. Heering, D. R. Weir, M. B. Ofstedal, and J. R. Burke, et al. 2007. "Prevalence of Dementia in the United States: The Aging, Demographics and Memory Study." *Neuroepidemiology* 29: 125–132.

Sabat, S. R. 1991. "Facilitating Conversation Via Indirect Repair: A Case Study of Alzheimer's Disease." *The Georgetown Journal of Languages and Linguistics* 2: 284–296.

Sabat, S. R. 1994. "Excess Disability and Malignant Social Psychology: A Case Study of Alzheimer's Disease." *Journal of Community and Applied Social Psychology* 4 (3): 157-166.

Sabat, S. R. 2001. *The Experience of Alzheimer's Disease: Life through a Tangled Veil.* Oxford: Blackwell.

Sabat, S. R. 2003. "Malignant Positioning and the Predicament of the Person with Alzheimer's Disease." In *The Self and Others: Positioning Individuals and Groups in Personal, Political, and Cultural Contexts.*, edited by F. M. Moghaddam and R. Harré, 85–98. Westport, CT: Greenwood Publishing Group, Inc.

Sabat, S. R. 2008. "A Bio-Psycho-Social Approach to Dementia." In *Excellence in Dementia Care: Research into Practice.*, edited by M. Downs and B. Bowers, 70–84. New York: Open University Press/McGraw Hill.

Sabat, S. R. 2012. "A Bio-Psycho-Social Model Enhances Young Adults' Understanding of and Beliefs About People with Alzheimer's Disease: A Case Study." *Dementia: The International Journal of Social Research and Practice* 11: 95–112.

Sabat, S. R., and M. Collins. 1999. "Intact Social, Cognitive Ability, and Selfhood: A Case Study of Alzheimer's Disease." *American Journal of Alzheimer's Disease* 14: 11–19.

Sabat, S. R., H. Fath, F. M. Moghaddam, and R. Harré. 1999. "The Maintenance of Self-esteem: Lessons from the Culture of Alzheimer's Sufferers." *Culture and Psychology* 5: 5–31.

Sabat, S. R., and C. M. Gladstone. 2010. "What Intact Social Cognition and Social Behavior Reveal About Cognition in the Moderate Stage of Alzheimer's Disease: A Case Study." *Dementia: The International Journal of Social Research and Practice* 9: 61–78.

Sabat, S. R., and R. Harré. 1992. "The Construction and Deconstruction of Self in Alzheimer's Disease." *Ageing and Society* 12: 443–461.

Sabat, S. R., and R. Harré. 1994. "The Alzheimer's Disease Sufferer as a Semiotic Subject." *Philosophy, Psychiatry, and Psychology* 1 (1): 145–160.

Sabat, S. R., and J. M. Lee. 2012. "Relatedness among People Diagnosed with Dementia: Social Cognition and the Possibility of Friendship." *Dementia: The International Journal of Social Research and Practice* 11: 311–323.

Sabat, S. R., L. Napolitano, and H. Fath. 2004. "Barriers to the Construction of a Valued Social Identity: A Case Study of Alzheimer's Disease." *American Journal of Alzheimer's Disease and Other Dementias* 19 (3): 177–185.

Shweder, R. A., and M. Sullivan. 1989. "The Semiotic Subject of Cultural Psychology." In *Handbook of Personality Theory and Research*, edited by L. Previn. New York: Guilford.

Stern, W. 1917. *Die Psychologie und der Personalismus* (Psychology and Personalism). Leipzig, Germany: Barth.

Stern, W. 1921. "Richtlinien für die Methodik der Psychologischen Praxis (Guidelines for the Method of Psychological Praxis)." *Beihefte zur Zeitschrift fur angewandte Psychologic* 29: 1–16.

Stern, W. 1923. *Person und Sache. System des Kritischen Personalismus. Band 2: Die Menschlische Personlichkeit* (Person and Thing: System of Critical Personalism. Volume 2: The Human Personality), 3rd unrevised edition. Leipzig, Germany: Barth.

Stern, W. 1929. "Personlichkeitsforschung und Testmethode (Personality Research and Testing Methods)." *Jahrbuch de Charakterologie* 6: 63–72.

Stern, W. 1938. *General Psychology from the Personalistic Standpoint*. Translated by H. D. Spoerl. New York: Macmillan. (Original work published in 1935.)

Ward, R., M. Howorth, H. Wilkinson, S. Campbell, and J. Keady. 2012. "Supporting the Friendships of People with Dementia." *Dementia: The International Journal of Social Research and Practice* 11: 287–303.

3

Dignity and Dementia: A Conceptual Exploration

LENNART NORDENFELT

Foreword

My purpose in this chapter is to explore the concept of dignity and its place in the care of the elderly and, in particular, in the care of persons with dementia. My presentation has a very specific point of departure. I was for four years involved in two projects, one of which was international, studying the dignity of older persons. The international project was supported by the European Commission and was called Dignity and Older Europeans (DOE) (the quality of life program QLG6-CT-2001-00888).

The DOE contained both theoretical and empirical studies. Among the theoretical studies was a philosophical analysis, performed by myself, partly in collaboration with Dr. Andrew Edgar, Cardiff University, of the basic concept of dignity. The main results of this analysis have already been published, for instance in *Dignity in Care for Older People* (Nordenfelt 2009). Here I start by presenting the model of dignity that we have proposed and continue by attempting to apply parts of the model to persons with dementia.

Introduction

In most medicolegal documents dignity is understood as the basic human dignity common to all mankind.[1] This is the dignity often referred to by the German word *Menschenwürde*, and this is the kind of dignity that has received most attention from contemporary philosophers. In this chapter, however, I contend that the language of dignity is much richer than this indicates. I intend to identify and explore four notions of dignity: (1) *Menschenwürde*, (2) the dignity of merit, (3) the dignity of moral stature, and (4) the dignity of identity.[2] I argue that they all play a role in our common Western discourse, in particular in the ethical discourse. The four notions indeed have a few elements in common. It is therefore perhaps more proper to talk of types of dignity, instead of notions of dignity. These elements, as I see them, are the following:

1. "Dignity" refers to a special dimension of value. In the case of *Menschenwürde* there is only one position on the scale, but with the other kinds people can have different positions on the scale; they can be more or less dignified.[3]
2. The dignity of a person is worthy of respect from others and from the person himself or herself.
3. The dignity has a ground, normally a set of properties, belonging to the subject.

In many but not all cases dignity attributes a set of rights to a person. Paying respect to dignity in these cases partly entails respecting the rights of the subject. But respect can also be expressed simply by thinking highly of the person or of the relevant qualities of the person.

The Four Concepts of Dignity

DIGNITY AS MERIT

A person who holds an office or has a rank that entails a set of rights has a special dignity. This is probably the oldest sense of the Latin *dignitas*, which was used to refer to excellence and distinction, properties typically pertaining to senators and other people of high rank in the Roman republic and the later empire. This is a sense that still flourishes in the Romance languages. The Spanish *dignidad* can refer to a person of a high rank, in particular in the clerical hierarchy, such as an archbishop.

We may refer to this dignity as dignity of merit, although in some cases a person may be born with such a dignity. Consider the case of a hereditary monarchy. Thus, for example, a king, a cabinet minister, a bishop, and a doctor have special dignities of merit that come with their positions. These are the *formal dignities of merit*. Typically, as the term implies, these dignities of merit are bestowed upon people through some formal act, for instance an appointment.

The dignity of merit is also related to the notions of rights and respect. The cabinet minister, the bishop, and the doctor have rights attached to their positions. These rights should be respected by those who approach the people in question.

It is significant that the dignities of merit can come and go. People can be promoted but they can also be demoted. People can for some time have an informal fame and a great reputation, but this can suddenly be gone. Another feature of the dignities of merit is that they admit of degrees. Many positions, professional or otherwise, are ordered in hierarchies. A general is higher on the military scale than a sergeant; a bishop is higher on the clerical scale than a prior.

DIGNITY AS MORAL STATURE

Let me now turn to a type of dignity that has some features in common with the general dignity of merit. It is a dignity of quite a special kind of merit: the dignity of moral stature. This is a dignity that is very much dependent upon the thoughts and deeds of the subject. We sometimes talk about a dignified character as a personality disposed to respect the moral law. Related to this is the idea that *dignified conduct* is action in accordance with the moral law.[4]

Sometimes the idea of dignified conduct is tied to actions of exceptional moral value, for instance in the face of extreme adversity and where the price paid is high. In extreme circumstances the price can be one's own life. Some famous historical persons did actually sacrifice their lives in order to preserve their dignity. One of these was the philosopher Socrates, who was sentenced to death for the alleged crime of having seduced the youth of Athens. In prison Socrates emptied a cup of poison and died in the company of some of his pupils. He thought that he would not have retained his dignity if he had fled from the prison, which in fact was quite possible for him (for a discussion of these cases, see Szawarski 1986, also Sulmasy 1997).

Like most ordinary dignities of merit, the dignity of moral stature is dimensional in that it can vary from an extremely high position to an extremely low one. Depending upon the moral value of one's actions, the degree of dignity is high or low. An important difference exists, however, between the dignities of merit and the dignity of moral stature in that the latter does not provide the subject with any rights. A prime minister has certain rights attached to the position held, so has the army general. But the extremely moral person has not acquired any rights through his or her deeds. It is an interesting feature of morality that the moral value of an action would be lost or at least diminished if the action were to result in certain rights or privileges for the subject.

THE DIGNITY OF IDENTITY

Let me now turn to a kind of dignity that is not dependent on the subject's merits, be they formal or informal, or having to do with the person's moral status. This kind of dignity is quite difficult to define. On the other hand this sense of dignity is probably the most important sense in the context of dignity and illness as well as the context of dignity and ageing. It is significant of this kind of dignity that it can be taken from us by external events, by the acts of other people as well as by injury, illness, and old age.

I call this *the dignity of identity*. It is the dignity that we attach to ourselves as integrated and autonomous persons, persons with a history and persons with a future, with all our relationships to other human beings.

Observe that I am not committing myself here to a particular theory of identity. I wish to keep the concept here as open as possible. What I refer to as identity may be narrated (or described) by myself and by others but, for my purposes, it need not be narrated by anybody. I would say that, for instance, a young child who does not yet have a language has an identity. A person with Alzheimer's disease (discussed later) also has an identity. Although these persons are normally described and their identity narrated by others, this is not presupposed by my concept of identity.

Most of us have a basic respect for our own identity, although this identity need not be at all remarkable from a moral or any other point of view. But this self-respect can easily be shattered, for instance by nature itself, in illness and the disability of illness and old age, but also by the cruel acts of other people.

Humiliation can be even more profound when it is the result of intentionally cruel acts. Statman (2000, 528) has reflected on this phenomenon in an insightful way:

> That other people can hit me, put me in jail and ridicule me publicly is beyond question. But why should such behaviors be taken as constituting a reason for me to respect myself less? How could it ever be rational to consider my *self*-respect injured because of the disrespect other people express toward me?

He goes on to say (534):

> Though the victim of humiliation often does not value the standards of worthiness and of social success assumed by the humiliator, the humiliator manages to shatter the victim's self-respect, to make her feel unworthy, diminished in stature, devalued.

There is a paradox here. How can humiliation rob me of my dignity? How can I lose my dignity when I am attacked by people whose moral views I despise? The humiliation is not (normally) a case of formal demotion. The perpetrators cannot (normally) do anything about my formal or informal merits. Nor can they by their immoral acts rob me of my moral stature. This can only happen if they succeed in provoking me to react in an immoral way.

So if there is a case of dignity here it is neither the dignity of merit nor the dignity of moral stature. It must be a dignity attached to the person's integrity and identity as a human being (see Kolnai 1976 for similar observations).

But is dignity in this sense, then, identical with a *feeling* or *sense* of worthiness? If we are only talking about a psychological fact (i.e., the self-confidence or self-respect of the person), then there is perhaps no need of a special concept of dignity.

I shall argue the case for an objective (or at least intersubjective) dignity of identity (cf. Edgar 2004). The cruel person can succeed in certain things apart from humiliating us. He or she can intrude into our private sphere, can physically hurt us, and can restrict our autonomy in many ways, for instance by putting us in jail. All these changes are extrapsychological. They do not just entail feelings of worthlessness or of humiliation. Intrusion in the private sphere is a violation of the person's integrity. Hurting a person is not only a violation of integrity; it also entails a change in the person's identity. The person is after this a person with a trauma; he or she has in a salient sense a new physical identity. The person's autonomy can be tampered with, when the person is prevented from doing what he or she wants to do or is entitled to do. Finally, insulting, hurting, or hindering somebody entails excluding this person from one's community.

Thus the factors that ground the dignity of identity are the subject's integrity and autonomy, including his or her social relations. These factors are typically associated with a sense of integrity and autonomy. When a person's integrity and autonomy are tampered with this is typically associated with a *feeling* of humiliation or loss of self-respect on his or her part. Self-respect is thus an important concept in connection also with the dignity of identity.

So far I have only considered the case where a person's self-respect has diminished or been lost as a result of another person's disrespectful acts. But the dignity of identity is relevant also in the cases when we say that illness, impairment, disability, and old age can rob one of one's dignity. What could happen in such cases?

To some extent we already have the answers. When one has had one's face badly damaged in a car accident, one's physical identity has been shattered. When, in the same kind of case, one has lost one's legs, one's physical identity is radically transformed and one's autonomy has been extremely diminished.[5]

A disabled person is almost per definition a person with restricted autonomy. Restricted autonomy normally entails exclusion from some communities.

Elderly people are often stricken with illness and disability. With the elderly there is an extra touch to this. Their disablement is often irreversible. The old person believes or knows that he or she will remain disabled for the rest of their life. The person's identity is for ever drastically changed.

THE DIGNITY OF *MENSCHENWÜRDE*

I have now introduced three notions of dignity, which are quite different but have two important features in common. First, people can have these types of dignity to various extents. Some people have high degrees of dignity, have a high rank in some hierarchy, have a high moral standard, and have an undamaged identity. Others score low along these dimensions and we can have combinations where a person has a high degree of dignity along one scale and a low one along another. Second, all three dignities can come and go. One can move from one position on a scale to another. One can be promoted at one time and demoted at another. One's moral status can rise and decline. One's identity can be shattered and restored. In particular with regard to the dignity of merit, one can even be completely removed from a scale and have no merit whatsoever.

In these important respects there is one kind of dignity that is completely different. The German word *Menschenwürde* refers to a kind of dignity that we all as humans have, or are assumed to have, just because we are humans. This is the specifically human value. We have this value to the same degree (i.e., we are equal with respect to this kind of dignity). It is significant that *Menschenwürde* cannot be taken from the human being as long as he or she is alive.

The idea of an equal human value is now common and accepted in the civilized world. It is a cornerstone in most religions and it has a strong place in Western secular ideology. The United Nations has attempted to capture this notion in its declaration of human rights. Let me quote from the *Universal Declaration of Human Rights* (1948). The first article states: "All human beings are born free, equal in dignity and human rights. They are endowed with reason and conscience and should act towards one another in a spirit of brotherhood."

But what is the ground for *Menschenwürde*? What is it about humans as a species that renders them a high dignity? One answer is the traditional monotheistic one: humans were created in God's image. The common modern answer, inspired by Kant, refers instead to capacities crucial to humans. The first is the human being's consciousness and ability to think (i.e., his or her reason). This includes the power of self-consciousness. Human beings can reflect upon themselves. Second, human beings are different from other creatures in the world through not being fixed. Human beings are free to decide their own way of life. Pico della Mirandola from the fifteenth century described how God the Father gave man an indeterminate nature ([1486] 1948, 227).

But if there is no predetermined goal in Nature, then the human being must also be the creator of norms and values. This is the third element in human dignity, viz. autonomy, most clearly explicated by Kant: "Autonomy is thus the basis of the dignity of both human nature and of every rational nature" ([1786] 1997, 53).

In short, *Menschenwürde* is a dignity belonging to every human being to the same degree all through his or her life. It cannot be taken away from any person and it cannot be attributed to any creature by fiat. The dignity of *Menschenwürde* is the ground for the specifically human rights.

Relations between the Notions of Dignity

It is interesting to inquire into the relationships between the various types of dignity that have been sketched here. Let me here look into the relation between the dignity of identity and *Menschenwürde*. How distinct are they and how important is it to distinguish between them? On the face of it they partly deal with the same matters. The reasons for protecting the dignity of identity seem to lie close to the reasons for protecting *Menschenwürde*. Moreover, both kinds of dignity are grounded on basic human properties, such as the conditions for life and autonomy.

It is also clear from my analysis that violating *Menschenwürde* is often tantamount to violating the dignity of identity. When *A* is cruel to *B* and does not respect *B*'s integrity then *A* violates *B*'s *Menschenwürde* and his or her dignity of identity. Conversely, respecting *Menschenwürde* is at the same time respecting a person's dignity of identity. What, then, is the reason for distinguishing between the two?

There are at least four features that distinguish *Menschenwürde* from dignity of identity and which I wish to underline here. The first two, and perhaps most crucial, are the ones mentioned in my summary above. *Menschenwürde* is fixed once and for all and it is the same for all people. The dignity of identity can vary between people and it can vary over time. The person who says, "I lost my dignity when my face was deformed in the car accident" must be talking of his or her dignity of identity. *Menschenwürde* can *ex hypothesi* not get lost.

A third distinguishing feature is embedded in my example above. *Menschenwürde*, like dignity of identity, can be violated by individuals and collectives of human beings, such as political parties and states. But *Menschenwürde*, unlike dignity of identity, cannot be violated by nature itself. However, a car accident and a natural phenomenon, in general, can rob a person of his or her dignity of identity. I highlighted earlier how diseases and the degenerating processes of old age can result in a deformation of a person's body and mind, with a reduction or even loss of dignity as a further result. Fourth, our common discourse suggests that even the dead can have a dignity that can be violated and tampered with. *Menschenwürde*, however, is *ex hypothesi* tied to the living human being.

The Relevance of the Four-notion Typology: How did the Interviewees Respond?

The question can now be asked: are the four types of dignity equally relevant in the context of care, be it ordinary health care or the care of the elderly and persons with dementia? My principal aim so far has been to make a basic and general analysis of the concepts of dignity. The fact that I mention the four types of dignity parallel to each other does not mean that I find them all to be equally relevant in health care or the care of the elderly and persons with dementia. It is clear from my presentations that *Menschenwürde* and dignity of identity are the two types that are most relevant in the context of care. This was also confirmed in the DOE study (Tadd and Calnan 2009). For older adults, it was, indeed, *Menschenwürde* and the dignity of identity that were most relevant. In the context of health and social care older people complained of being ignored, of being treated as objects, of having their need for privacy insufficiently recognized, of being humiliated and ridiculed, and of inappropriate forms of address being used. The neglect of privacy has had an impact on the dignity of identity and centered on various situations involving toileting; intimate care being delivered by members of the opposite sex, especially in the case of older women; or being moved on a hoist with intimate body parts on display.

The dignity of moral stature was also relevant, but in a different way from the others. The professionals thought that one should require a high moral status from the *provider* of the care. The provider should act morally (i.e., in a dignified way). There is, for natural reasons, not the same requirement with regard to the patients themselves. Professionals also reported their frustration at being unable to live up to the moral and professional requirements of their role, due to a lack of resources, under-staffing, or inadequate care environments.

Elements of dignity of merit came to the fore in the interviews, but normally in a negative way. To experience dignity of merit an individual has to be recognized by society as having dignity, and many older people thought that they were not recognized or valued in modern society, making this type of dignity difficult to experience. The dignity of merit was also discussed by young and middle-aged adults in terms of its impact on the individual's self-esteem and in relation to the impact of inadequate finances on social inclusion.

Dignity, the Elderly, and Persons with Dementia

Let me now turn to the more specific question whether there is a special dignity attached to elderly people or people with dementia. Is there such a dignity, or why should we otherwise pay special attention to them? Or, do any of the mentioned varieties of dignity apply more significantly to them? This is of particular importance when we deal with elderly people who are at the same time persons with dementia.

Let me first point to *Menschenwürde* as the basic platform. Every elderly person has his or her intrinsic basic value, which entails a number of rights, among others the rights of the UN declaration. The elderly person does not lose any of these rights because he or she has reached a particular age or is affected by a serious illness. It is a different matter that a few of the rights do not apply to the elderly because of their age, for instance the right to a proper school education or the right to work. But this does not distinguish the elderly from infants. Other basic rights, on the other hand, have greater application to the elderly, for instance, the universal right to care in the case of illness or disability.

Menschenwürde covers a great deal when it comes to paying respect to the dignity of the elderly and persons with dementia. This value is indeed, in spite of its basic position in all our philosophies of man, worth emphasizing, since it is in practice so often violated, not least in institutions for the elderly. A reason behind such violation may be the relatively low public status that the elderly and people with dementia have in many circles, in particular among the very young. *Menschenwürde* does not, however, cover the whole area of dignity relevant to the elderly or persons with dementia. I will in the following in particular focus on the dignity of identity.

A CHARACTERIZATION OF PERSONS WITH DEMENTIA

In the description of dementia a salient feature is often loss of ability. Persons suffering from dementia gradually lose their ability to orient themselves in time and space, suffer memory losses, and in particular lose their ability to communicate. They can act in ways that may be understood as irrational or even absurd. In short, persons with dementia present behavior deviating from that of the vast majority of humans, and from what is considered to be ideal or desirable for a human being.

Thus persons with dementia can be said to have lost a part of their former identity. They are now partly different persons than before. They are not as autonomous as before, they have lost some of their communicative capacity, but as we also know, practically never *all* communicative capacity.

Franklin, Ternestedt, and Nordenfelt (2006) have particularly investigated this phenomenon in an interview study of elderly nursing home residents, some of whom were in an early stage of dementia. A strong experience among these elderly people was that they were no longer able to control their functions. This recognition was a threat to their self-image and identity. "Losing different bodily functions meant an almost inevitable dependency that the elderly people experienced as violating and difficult to handle despite their reconciliation with their situation on another level" (138).

A common consequence of such disabilities related to old age and dementia is that people around the elderly change their attitudes toward them.

> You see...it feels as if they treat us as if we don't understand anything even though we have lived a whole life. (Franklin et al. 2006, 139)

In the case of certain people with dementia there is often also a remarkable change in their looks. For some people this marks an extremely painful change of identity. The beautiful woman, whose identity has largely consisted of her beauty, is through age and illness gradually transformed into a much less attractive person. Likewise, the athlete, whose fame was wholly dependent on achievements on the track, is over time gradually transformed into a weak, disabled person who is excluded from the community of the old days.

Disability and restricted autonomy have a further consequence for a person's identity and thereby dignity. Persons with dementia and the old who cannot move about and take care of themselves are relegated to other people—their caretakers. The risk of intrusion into one's private sphere (i.e., of a violation of one's integrity) then becomes high.

What has happened to these persons' *dignity* of identity? At an early stage they would often themselves describe their situation as entailing a certain loss of dignity. This is similar to the situation for many persons with other illnesses. They would say that nature has deprived them of a part of their dignity. They cannot any longer do what they wish and they cannot fulfil their earlier potential. But this does not mean that there is no identity left and that there is no *dignity* of identity. In many ways the persons with dementia are gifted persons; they are persons with a complex inner life. They have retained some memories; they have never, if they are at all conscious, lost all memories. This can be shown in many ways, by the recognition of other people and by the recognition of phenomena around them, not least phenomena that are related to early and emotionally loaded events.

We have discussed older people in general and persons with mild and moderate forms of dementia. But now let us turn to the more extreme cases of people with severe dementia, where it is not only a question of loss of physical abilities and loss of memory but also a question of severe loss of mental abilities to the extent that the subjects cannot express themselves in ordinary language and cannot even recognize their nearest and dearest.

I would suggest that the philosophy of Merleau-Ponty (1945/1962) provides us with intellectual tools to analyze such situations. Following Merleau-Ponty one can argue that the subjectivity of the human being is not limited to cases where there is self-consciousness or a specific degree of conscious awareness. A sleeping person is still a subject. A person in a coma is still a subject. "Even in sleep and in a coma, the lived body is still 'constituting meaning', although this level of meaning is not the meaning we traditionally refer to when we speak about meaning" (Bullington 2009, 72).

These observations have an obvious bearing on the case of persons of dementia, even severe dementia. Such persons may have peculiar, even idiosyncratic, ways of expressing themselves. They cannot always express their experiences, intentions, and desires in words. But—and this is important—the communication can be performed in body language, by behavior that often expresses emotions, emotions of love, friendship, suspiciousness, anger, or fear.

Professor Eric Matthews (2006, 175) argues in this direction in a very insightful way. He provides the following example:

> An example that comes to my mind is that of an elderly woman with dementia I know of, who recalls little of her past life and is barely aware of where she is now. Nevertheless, one part of her past that she still retains is her ingrained sense of politeness, which is expressed in certain of her spontaneous ways of behaving.

Here Matthews describes a woman with a salient personality, an identity, although this personality does not at all have the completeness of her self in earlier days. She is still certainly a body-subject in Merleau-Ponty's sense. She reacts intentionally, in a way that is typical for her, to a common situation in life. She is easily to be recognized as the person she once was. She has a dignity of identity, which may be somewhat diminished now, but still exists.

It is interesting to add that this particular person also has a significant dignity of moral standing. The trait she displays in the situations described by Matthews is a trait of morality. She is polite and considerate in relation to people around her. Her politeness is certainly intentional and not mechanical.

THE WISDOM OF ELDERLY PEOPLE

In an earlier publication (Nordenfelt 2009) I made the point, with regard to older people, that they possess a particular variant of dignity of merit. I call this variant the *dignity of wisdom*. What, then, do I mean by wisdom?

Wisdom is a kind of knowledge; it is not, however, just the simple knowledge of a fact, or even the complicated knowledge of a scientific system. Wisdom is knowledge whose object is life, more specifically *human* life. The wise person knows what life is like in general. The wise person also understands the complications of life. But wisdom is also practical knowledge in the sense that the wise know what to do in a particular situation, mainly because the wise have already experienced a similar situation (cf. Aristotle's notion of *phronesis*, which entails the skill to apply ethical principles to individual cases). The wise person must to some extent be a moral person. I doubt, however, that we should identify the wise with the moral. I trace a fascinating element in wisdom that is such that the wise may sometimes challenge morality, at least traditional morality.

By definition older people have all lived a long life. They have a long experience of the various hardships and blessings in life. They know what life is all about. All this is a necessary part, but probably not the whole, of the crucial virtue of *wisdom*. My conjecture, then, is that all elderly people have the dignity of merit of wisdom. This conjecture is not original. For some cultures—particularly prominent examples are the cultures of China and Japan—this assumption is a cornerstone. On the basis of the ancient Confucian teachings the elderly have always been treated with much reverence and care in these countries. (For a thorough analysis of the Chinese situation, see for instance Engelhardt 2007.)

As I indicated above, a long life's experience, with all its necessary ingredients of education, work, love, frustrated love, disappointments, grief at death, illness, but also quite often of blessings of partnership and children, gives a good ground for wisdom, to many people a sufficient ground. But does it not entail, one may ask, some endowment, although not a remarkable one, to digest these experiences in a proper way, so that wisdom arises? Can we not suspect and do we not know that some people do not have this minimal endowment? About some people we sometimes use the locution: they will never learn.

I certainly grant that there is a difference between people in this respect. It is not just empty to say that some people are really wise and that some are not wise at all, or at least they do not display their wisdom. So, if we accept that all elderly people are wise in some way, they must be wise to different degrees. Some elderly people have experienced more variety in life, a few have even experienced extreme horrors, whereas others have lived an extremely uniform and sheltered life. Some elderly people have more intellectual and emotional gifts than others. This means that some of the elderly have had more ability to learn from life than others. Thus their wisdom cannot be equal.

It is tempting to say in our context that the persons with grave dementia must be the ones who are the least wise among humans. Their intellectual abilities are severely damaged and they may have little potential to show their awareness of what is happening to them. Can we reasonably ascribe wisdom to them?

I think that the Merleau-Pontian argument put forward above has a bearing also in this context. Certainly, the person with severe dementia cannot be called a wise person in the full-blown sense. But there may be quite strong wise fragments left. The emotional self may still be quite strong. Persons with dementia may be quite able to detect when there is a conflict between people close to them and they may express their grief at this. They may also, like the woman described by Matthews, have kept their strong moral attitude and display it on appropriate occasions. One could perhaps say, using Merleau-Ponty's wording, that there is some wisdom sedimented in the unconscious structure of the body of the person with dementia. Thus there is wisdom here that should be acknowledged and revered.

Notes

1. See, for instance, Council of Europe 1997.
2. A presentation of the four types of dignity has appeared earlier in Nordenfelt 2004 and more developed in Nordenfelt 2009.
3. For a valuable analysis of the semantics of dignity, see Kolnai 1976.
4. Some theorists (including Kolnai 1976) have convinced me that there is a further sense of the expression "dignified behavior," which refers rather to the aesthetic than the moral properties of the behavior in question. These are, for instance, qualities that have to do with composure, calmness, and restraint.
5. Autonomy is here understood in the theoretical sense of "having the power" to perform a certain action.

References

Bullington, Jennifer. 2009. "Being Body: The Dignity of Human Embodiment." In *Dignity in Care for Older People*, edited by Lennart Nordenfelt. Oxford: Wiley-Blackwell.

Council of Europe. 1997. *Convention for the Protection of Human Rights and Dignity of the Human Being With Regard to the Application of Biology and Medicine: Convention on Human Rights and Medicine*. Strasbourg: European Treaty Series No.164.

Dignity and Older Europeans. 2004. *Final Report of Focus Groups (2002–2004)*. http://www.cardiff.ac.uk/socsi/dignity/europe/index.html. Accessed on August 22, 2012.

Edgar, Andrew. 2004. "A Response to Nordenfelt's 'The Varieties of Dignity'." *Health Care Analysis* 12: 83–89.

Engelhardt, H. Tristram Jr. 2007. "Long-Term Care: The Family, Post-Modernity, and Conflicting Moral Life-Worlds." *The Journal of Medicine and Philosophy* 32: 519–536.

Franklin, Lise-Lotte, Britt-Marie Ternestedt, and Lennart Nordenfelt. 2006. "Views on Dignity of Elderly Nursing Home Residents." *Nursing Ethics* 13: 1–15.

Kant, Immanuel. 1997. *Foundations of the Metaphysics of Morals*. Translated by L.W. Beck. Upper Saddle River, NJ: Prentice Hall.

Kolnai, Aurel. 1976. "Dignity." *Philosophy* 51: 251–271.

Matthews, Eric. 2006. "Dementia and the Identity of the Person." In *Dementia: Mind, Meaning and the Person*, edited by Julian C. Hughes, Stephen J. Louw, and Steven R. Sabat. Oxford: Oxford University Press.

Merleau-Ponty, Maurice. 1945/1962. *Phenomenology of Perception*. London: Routledge & Kegan Paul.

Nordenfelt, Lennart. 2004. "The Varieties of Dignity." *Health Care Analysis* 12: 69–81.

Nordenfelt, Lennart. 2009. "The Concept of Dignity." In *Dignity in Care for Older People*, edited by Lennart Nordenfelt. Oxford: Wiley-Blackwell.

Pico della Mirandola, Giovanni. 1948. "On the Dignity of Man." In *The Renaissance Philosophy of Man*, edited by Ernst Cassirer, Paul Oskar Kristeller, and John Herman Randall. Chicago: The University of Chicago Press, Chicago.

Statman, Daniel. 2000. "Humiliation, Dignity and Self-Respect." *Philosophical Psychology* 13: 523–540.

Sulmasy, Daniel P. 1997. "Death With Dignity: What Does It Mean?" *Josephinum Journal of Theology* 4: 13–23.

Szawarski, Zbigniew. 1986. "Dignity and Responsibility." *Dialectics and Humanism* 2-3: 193–205.

Tadd, Winifred and Michael Calnan. 2009. "Care for Older People: Why Dignity Matters—the European Experience." In *Dignity in Care for Older People*, edited by Lennart Nordenfelt. Oxford: Wiley-Blackwell.

United Nations. 1948. *The Universal Declaration of Human Rights*, adopted and proclaimed by General Assembly resolution 217 A (111) of 10 December 1948. Geneva: The Office of the High Commissioner for Human Rights.

4

"I'm his wife not his carer!"—Dignity and Couplehood in Dementia

INGRID HELLSTRÖM

"Our two selves"

> Well, she was gone now. I could not be the person I had been; the one who was part of her when she died of Alzheimer's disease. She had taken our two selves with her. I could see my old self clearly enough, but only as a fact of history, unrelated to what I seemed to have become. (Bayley 2001, 4)

John Bayley[1] writes about his late wife, Dame Iris Murdoch, the famous British novelist and philosopher, during her Alzheimer's disease. In a trilogy[2] Bayley has in a very honest way described their more than forty years of marriage, their time together during Murdoch's Alzheimer's disease, and his own experiences of being a widower. He writes that Murdoch had taken their "two selves" with her when she died, his and hers. Even though they as individuals were described by Bayley (1998, 1999, 2001) as very independent, they were at the same time during their marriage always a couple, a unit.

This chapter is devoted to older husbands and wives living with dementia who in different ways try to sustain their couplehood and balance their actions in everyday life in order not to humiliate their partner. The concept of couplehood is in this context something more than the sum of two individuals and should be looked upon as a phenomenon that could take different forms over time and could be influenced in various ways. The chapter is mainly based on data from a longitudinal interview study with twenty spouses living with dementia (Hellström, Nolan, and Lundh 2007). The aim of the study was to explore the ways in which older people with dementia and their spouses experience dementia over time, especially the impact it had on their interpersonal relationships and patterns of everyday life. At inclusion the spouses were 65–85 years old and had been living together for between eight and sixty years, the majority more than fifty years. The concept of dignity was one of the themes brought up during the repeated interviews, which were conducted for up to five years, on five to six occasions.

Dignity is a multifaceted concept (Moody 1998, 23) and some have questioned if it should be used at all in ethical analysis in health care (Macklin 2003, 1419). Others, for example Leget (2012), emphasize that dignity is vague but argue that for it to be useful one must account for the different types of the concept. Pullman (1999, 35) makes a distinction between basic and personal dignity. Basic dignity should not be reduced in any way, regardless of various attributes pertaining to the individual person, for example a specific occupation or illnesses. Personal dignity, however, is socially constructed and can be influenced in different degrees. Nordenfelt (2009, 40) differentiates between four types of dignity: (1) human dignity, (2) dignity of merit, (3) dignity of moral stature, and (4) dignity of identity. Human dignity refers to a specific human value that remains undiminished as long as a person is alive; it relates to Pullman's (1999) notion of basic dignity. Dignity of merit relates to the dignity bestowed by reason of rank or standing. The dignity of moral stature relates to self-respect, and concerns the respect people have for themselves as moral human beings.

The focus in this chapter is on the dignity of identity, which according to Nordenfelt relates to a person's integrity, autonomy, life history, and relationships with other people. This dignity may vary depending on the attitude of others toward an individual, and consequently is influenced by changes to an individual's body and mind (Nordenfelt 2009, 33). Elderly persons with dementia are at risk of losing such dignity, but what of couples living with dementia, couples who look upon themselves as a unit consisting of "two selves"? Is there a risk of losing a *shared* dignity of identity?

Being "chained to a corpse"

Traditionally, people with dementia were thought to eventually lose their selves (Basting 2003, 88) and to be transformed to an "unbecoming self" with the "body unimpaired" (Fontana and Smith 1989, 36); however, nowadays, this view is questioned (Caddel and Clare 2010, 124). The negative images of ageing and old age in Western society that we have today developed during the nineteenth century when there was an interest in describing ageing and old age systematically in the medical literature (Kirk 1995, 288). There is also a discourse of a "second childhood" and older people are sometimes referred as "going ga-ga" (the utterance "ga-ga" is also used in Swedish in the expression "*gaggig*"). Hockey and James write that "through this mutual referencing, old age is drawn into alignment with dependency of early childhood" (1993, 17).

People with dementia are not only exposed to the negative images of old age, but also to the negative images of the dementia diagnosis itself. A "decline paradigm" prevails (Dunham and Cannon 2008, 46). For example, Alzheimer's disease is reframed as "the dread disease afflicting an ageing society" (Ballenger 2008, 495) and it seems that older, cognitively intact people fear dementia (Corner and Bond 2004, 153).

In descriptions of a life with dementia, negative stereotyping is common (Scholl and Sabat 2008), as are negative metaphors. People with dementia are compared to zombies (Behuniak 2011, 85) or the disease is compared to an epidemic (e.g., you can catch it), an enemy soldier, or a predatory thief (e.g., it creeps up) (Johnstone 2011, 6–10)—I know of no metaphors with a more positive connotation. Furthermore, we live in a culture where cognitive function has a high value (Post 1995) and it is important to be able to recognize your relatives, or more precisely to tell facts about them, otherwise they are likely to think you are "lost" or experiencing a "social death" (Taylor 2008, 322). As Post puts it, "It is easy to be against people with dementia because our culture is against forgetfulness" (1995, 2).

These negative images not only have an impact on the person with dementia, they also could influence how spouses describe their own caregiving. Bayley (1998) compared his own experience in contradistinction with the experience of a lady he had met during the time of Murdoch's illness. He writes:

> The lady who told me in her own deliberately jolly way that living with an Alzheimer victim was like being chained to a corpse, went on to an ever greater access of desperate facetiousness. "And, as you and I know, it's a corpse that complains all the time." I don't know it. In spite of her anxious and perpetual queries Iris seems not to know how to complain. She never has. Alzheimer's, which can accentuate personality traits to the point of demonic parody, has only been able to exaggerate a natural goodness in her. (Bayley 1998, 83–84)

Just as people with dementia are at great risk of being seen as having lost their selves (Basting 2003) so too the spouse loses his or her spousal identity and is transformed to a caregiver.

In the following I describe how three elderly men with dementia (Hans, Lars, and Karl) and their wives (Maria, Lisa, and Eva), all with different living conditions, tried to create a "nurturative relational context" (Hellström, Nolan, and Lundh 2007, 390) in order to sustain their couplehood. These couples differ from each other in various ways. One example was the different degrees of mobility. Hans and Maria were both very active and had no physical impairments. They were able to travel and, in adjusted form, to continue with their former interests. In the case of Lars and Lisa, Lisa was physically impaired and dependent on support from home service. This couple seldom left their home. In the third couple, Karl and Eva, Karl was physically impaired in addition to his dementia. As with the case of Lars and Lisa, this third couple seldom left their home together because of Karl's dementia. Eva had to go out alone. This was only one aspect of different conditions for couples living with dementia, yet it had an impact on their *shared* dignity of identity, on their integrity, autonomy, life story, and relationships with other people.

"I'm being reflected"

The first couple, Hans and Maria, had been living together for forty-five years. They met during a ski holiday in northern Sweden. Since then, they have both taken part in various leisure activities and their great interest was to travel abroad. In his late sixties, Hans was diagnosed having Alzheimer's disease and he was convinced that his symptoms started during a trip to Kenya, when he fell ill with a stomach virus at their hotel. Maria had another view about how they both became aware of his memory problems, but she never dwelled on this subject. At the time of the first interview Hans was seventy-two years old and his wife seventy. They lived in a big house, with a patio, in a small community.

Hans and Maria were almost always together and did things together. One thing they did together was go bowling. At the time of the fourth interview Hans visited a day care center twice a week. Maria had her own activities on these days, but on Fridays they played together with their friends. She said:

> There are not so many [participants] there on Fridays so it usually goes pretty well. They also know about it [his Alzheimer's disease], those who are there. I always tell them to help Hans, because we do not play the same team every time.... But he throws well and is participating, but he has no idea who will win or lose or anything. But it does not matter; he takes part in all the cases. It is in this way that we have to do the kinds of activities that we both can participate in.

They were very active in the community, where they had lived since late 1960s. For example, they took part in a choir that performed in nursing homes, helped older and physically impaired people to spend some time outside their caring facilities, and practiced folk dance. Additionally, Hans was interested in ornithology and used to walk in the forest by himself. However, after an incident when he got lost, he promised Maria that he would not take a walk without company. He thought that it was no problem, but out of consideration for his wife he tried to remember this promise, even though he forgot it sometimes. Hans showed that he could imagine how his wife would feel if he was lost again and he did not want to expose her to this.

> No, I don't do it [take walk on my own]. It happened once, earlier this spring or what you should say, eh, we went to the forest and then I sort of went away, Maria you see, she started to look for me and we missed one other in some way, I don't know, then it was some sort of crisis you see, I didn't find it that dangerous, myself, it was worse for her.

At the second interview Maria explained that:

> If I'm sort of harmonious and like this it has an impact on him you see, then he also is as well, he mirrors himself in me all the time, I can't have a bad temper, irritated or like that, I can't...I do small things now and then and then we have time for activities and we have time for a ride on our bicycles and then we have time for a rest.

The way she acted was reflected in the way that Hans reacted. He was mirroring her. Hans was well aware that Maria sometimes lost her patience with him and he tried to avoid situations that could upset her. She also said that it was important that she tried to be calm because he was "reflecting himself in her." She knew that she had to rest to be able to support him, and if she needed to rest during the day, her husband sat quietly beside her on the bed and waited for her.

She tried to be and look patient, and she made an effort to find assignments in the home for him that he could manage on his own. When he tried to do things in the home, like cleaning the bathroom, he realized that he was not up to it and became very distressed. He often cried on these occasions. The wife said that she hugged him and tried to talk about other things, and this often worked. He liked very much to sit beside his wife, holding her hand. However, he disliked when she read her books because she was not present in the degree he wished; he was, in other words, not able to interpret what she was experiencing.

He also thought that his memory problems had a greater impact on his wife because she was the one who had to take care of everything. Sometimes things got worse when he tried to help her out, for example, in the kitchen. He said in the third interview:

> I: Do you think that it [memory problems] has an impact on Maria's everyday life?
> Hans: Yes, it does, oh yes, it's worse for her I think.
> I: Hhm
> Hans: I think anyway, it ought to be I think, I, sort of, can't do anything to help out, it's almost worse if I'm going to do something.

Maria described this in almost the same way: "He wants to do so much, and sometimes I set him to doing something then, something simple. But it becomes crazy. It would be much better if I did it myself."

At the time of the last interview Hans had moved into a group home for people with dementia. Maria visited him several times a week, and even though she still was very active with different activities with their friends, she said that she missed him all the time. Hans had an advanced aphasia at that moment, and Maria was the only one who was able to interpret parts of what he was telling her. She also tried to do things that they both could enjoy; they tried to sustain their relationship beyond words. They took walks in the city together and they also danced in his apartment at the group home. This was a way for the couple to sustain not only their relationship but also a common interest, folk dance. However, their experience of reality did not always agree. Hans thought they had an audience looking at them from the sofa or from his pictures on the wall. Maria said that he should not bother, just enjoy the moment.

> Maria: Sometimes, I dance with him because he loves dancing.
> I: Yes.
> Maria: And we dance here [meaning his apartment], there is a lot of space and then he says "Oh, they [people on the sofa or in pictures] sit there and they laugh at us!" "Yes, let them laugh, they have a fun moment as well."

Maria explained in the interview that Hans felt very safe at his group home and did not actually express any fear for "the people on the sofa or in the pictures"; he just seemed a bit embarrassed by the fact that they danced in front of an audience. In sum, this couple presented their shared life story and integrity as being very close. Hans was never, during the course of the study, physically impaired, and Maria never let their relationships with other people be affected to any greater extent. She tried always to adjust to Hans's impairment and in the way he "reflected himself in her."

"One is the head, the other one the legs"

The daily life of Lars and Lisa could be characterized as being more circumscribed compared to the life of Maria and Hans. The couple lived in a modern apartment. Earlier they had lived in a villa in the same area of the town. Lisa was seventy-three years old and Lars was seventy-six years old and they had been living together for forty-nine years. The couple had two daughters, one of which supported her parents every other day at the beginning of the study. At one point in time there was some sort of disagreement between the daughter and her father so she did not visit them as often as she used to. There was also a disagreement between the two daughters as to how to handle their father and how to support their parents.

During the repeated interviews Lars stressed that he and his wife Lisa always helped each other. He had Alzheimer's disease while his wife had severe rheumatic disease and was dependent on her wheelchair to move around in the apartment. For example, she was not able to lift her arms above her shoulders and therefore not able to fetch china from the kitchen cupboard, or collect things from the floor she had dropped. Lars said at the first interview:

> It's everything that we have each other and help each other. We are both handicapped in this way, in different ways. One has the head [meaning his wife] and the other one has the legs [meaning himself]

This couple could be characterized as a vulnerable dyad (Hermansson 1990, 16), which signifies a couple that is almost independent as long as they stay together. Lisa often was very tired, both as a result of her own disease, and as a result of Lars' Alzheimer's disease and his penchant for losing things and stubbornness. Despite this, she admitted that she would not have been able to live alone in the apartment. Lisa had to stay calm and expressed pride over the fact that she usually could handle conflicts between herself and Lars and also within their close family. For example, for some period of time Lars was convinced that he did not need to take a bath or change his clothes regularly. That meant that there was a constant smell around him and during this time Lisa avoided inviting people to their home. She knew that there was no point in nagging him because it would only make him upset and sometimes angry. He looked upon himself as if it was he who supported her with practical chores in their home, not the opposite, even though he agreed that he had memory problems and needed to be reminded of different things. At the beginning of the study, the couple only had a safety alarm connected to the home help service, but over time they started to use home help and meal delivery on a regular basis. However, Lisa had to introduce these services very slowly, one small task at a time, because her husband did not agree that they needed help. He thought that the home helpers were taking away his role of supporting his wife.

Lisa was dependent on him, in spite of the home helpers who visited them several times a day. Lars was dependent on her to live at home. However, he sometimes forgot that he had promised to help her whenever she needed him. During the night it was hard for him to handle the situation. Lisa said during the fourth interview:

> It's so funny, because every evening when we go to bed he says "You just tell me tonight if you need help, it's nothing, I wake up and then a go to sleep again." But when you are at this specific situation yes, no, it was not so good right then, then he had forgotten that too.

Lisa was a bit reluctant to leave the apartment with Lars. She explained that Lars was not capable of handling dangerous situations. For example, because of his dementia, he had difficulty judging the distance between the pavement and the street. Lisa explained:

> I: Do you leave [the apartment] together, or—?
> Lisa: We used to before. I hardly dare, Lars cannot handle the wheelchair, it has worked fine, but sometimes he is so close to the edge so that I'm almost afraid it will go downhill, and it's not so funny either to sit and be anxious then, but we'll see this summer. Then, if nothing else, we can sit on the balcony so that we come out and we see people there.

Instead of going out together with Lars, Lisa tried to find out things that were meaningful for her husband. Lars liked to talk about his childhood and nowadays he spent time organizing pictures of his family, letters, and other documents connected to his life story. Lisa spent a lot of time listening to his stories; some of them she had heard several times before.

This vulnerable couple stayed indoors most of the time, depending on Lars's Alzheimer's disease as well as on Lisa's physical impairment, and that had an influence on their ability to have a relationship with other people. Additionally, there were some disagreements within their close family. For Lars, the interest in his life story was prominent, and Lisa seemed to adjust to this fact. She never expressed openly during the interviews that she wished to talk about their shared life story, or about her own, simply that Lars focused on his. Lars had difficulty grasping that he sometimes needed support with, for example, his personal hygiene. He seemed not to be willing to let anyone into his personal sphere. Lisa adjusted to this as well and just stayed calm and waited for him to change his mind.

"I don't treat him like a child"

In the last case we turn to Karl and Eva. At the first interview Karl was eighty years old and his wife Eva sixty-eight years of age. They had been living together for almost forty years. This was Karl's second marriage and he had a son, with whom he had no contact. Their closest next of kin was Eva's older brother, who lived in the neighborhood. The couple lived in a small cottage in the countryside, which on one side faced wide fields and on the other side a forest. The cottage consisted of a living room, a small kitchen, and a small bedroom. The bathroom was situated in the basement. Karl was diagnosed having mixed dementia and two of his more prevalent symptoms were his memory problems and his lack of orientation in time. However, if asked, he had no problem telling facts about his life and his areas of interest, for example rock climbing, car racing, and names of birds and flowers. Before his retirement he had, among other things, had a position as a construction worker. He was the one who had built their cottage. Eva presented her husband, at every interview, as if he had been a strong and competent person:

> Karl was one of those people who worked outside, he was making the fire in the boiler, huh, he took wood in the forest and chopped and I wondered how on earth he manage to lift that wood, but he kept on until, well not last year he could not, because he had so much pain in his knee, but I think he is a man who is used to being outside.

Eva mentioned pain in his knee, and at the time of the interviews Karl was dependent on his wheelchair to move around in the cottage and in their garden. In addition to his dementia he had had an accident and hurt his right leg badly; he became physically impaired. To support his everyday life, the couple had received different aids that occupied large parts of the bedroom. As a result, there was no room for Eva's bed and she had to sleep on the sofa in their hall. In an attempt to sustain their relationship, Eva had declined help from the home service in the morning; as long as it was possible she wanted to manage on her own. The mornings belonged to them. She explained that in the early mornings she brought him tea and some bread and then she sat beside him in his bed and they looked at the morning television together. That meant that Karl stayed in his bed most of the morning, but the bed was also his "safe place," and he was pleased when he spent time there. It was also the only time in the day when Eva could leave the house for a couple of hours. During his illness he had started to be afraid of different things, for example, moving from the bed into his wheelchair, going by car, looking at dangerous animals on the television. Eva had tried to introduce an electric wheelchair so he would be able to move around in their surroundings, but she explained that it was too scary for him, he preferred his old chair. At the fourth interview Karl needed a lot of help from the interviewer to focus on the different topics and he explained about his wheelchairs:

> I: It works well with the wheelchair and so? [the interviewer is clapping on the armrest on his wheelchair]
> Karl: Yes, of course. It's part of it all, you know. She [Eva] is running it.
> I: Have you used the electric wheelchair this summer?
> Karl: No, it stays there [in their garage].
> I: Was it hard to use, or?
> Karl: No.
> I: You are happy with this one?
> Karl: Yes it's ok. It has forward and reverse.

As illustrated above, Karl had rather serious difficulties in everyday life. He was in a way totally dependent on his wife Eva and on the home help service. Eva explained that when she was working in the garden, he used to call to her and urge her to be careful with herself. She was also aware of the fact that Karl was very sensitive to being treated "like a child." She had seen that some of the home helpers treated him in this way. She did not like it, but tried not to mind because she was also dependent on their support in the evenings or when Karl needed to take a bath, as he was too heavy for her to manage on her own. In contrast to the formal caregivers, she was determined to treat him like he was her husband, not her child. She said:

> But you don't want to let it go and think, "Now I will treat him like a child," that I could not do. You want him to keep—his dignity, yes dignity or whatever you want to call it, and treat him as [I did] before, then, then [I] manage to do it up to a point, but then you become angry.

Although they sometimes had their quarrels, she pushed him to take part in different decisions, "simple stuff," as she called it, but she thought it was vital for him. Some days Karl got the idea that, for example, he needed to get ready to go to work. On these occasions Eva tried to have a discussion with him about what retirement means, and as she said, "*I want him to think.*" And she preferred him to be confident in his own abilities rather than have low self-confidence:

> I: How do you handle the situation when he wants to go to work?
> Eva: But you know, he is, I mean he has difficulties moving you know, so that's nothing, I just say "But please, Karl, luckily we are both retired

you see, so you don't have to go to work," then I ask, because I really like him to think, I want him to think "Is it really possible," to think. Then I say that "You have a stiff leg, how could you manage to work, what type of job will you do?" I want him to think rationally about what I say, but it's not that easy every time.

Eva also adjusted different tasks for him at home as ways of helping Karl feel that he was valuable. At the time of the first interview, Karl had managed, sitting in his wheelchair, to prune the apple trees in their garden while Eva collected the branches. He also took care of the heating in their cottage, sitting in his wheelchair. At the last interview he was assigned a more undemanding task, wiping the cutlery when Eva did the washing up, even though he was not able to put the cutlery back in the right order. Eva did not mind rearranging it later on. But for him it was important to help his wife with at least one chore in their household. Eva also started to notice that their old friends had begun to avoid talking to Karl, and observed that younger people found it easier to listen to Karl's stories. She felt that she could manage both the physical and psychological strain, but one thing made her sad—that their common life story was in danger of being lost. They had no children and she had no one to discuss the life story with. Karl had started to forget large parts of their shared life and she was solely responsible for preserving it.

To sum up, in the three cases described it could easily be seen that the couples handled their "*shared dignity*" in different ways depending on their different life stories and living conditions. Dignity seemed to be interrelated between the two members of the couple; humiliation of one spouse often meant humiliation of the couple as a unit. In the case of Karl and Eva, Eva was very careful not to treat her husband as a child. She seemed to be well aware of the discourse of second childhood, even though it was not explicitly expressed (Hockey and James 1993, 17). Eva presented Karl as strong person, not as a child. We can only speculate here, but if she had presented him as a child she would have been regarded herself as a mother to her own husband. Instead she tried to sustain their couplehood in an adjusted form, for example by having tea in his bed each morning. Another example is Lars, even though he did not care for his own hygiene for a period of time, it was Lisa who withdrew from socialization with other people in order not to expose, not only Lars, but also herself from being positioned as filthy. She felt responsible for Lars' actions. Lars had difficulties letting someone into his personal sphere, but on the other hand he looked upon himself with dignity as he helped Lisa with her hygiene and with her clothes. That was the reason Lisa introduced the home help very slowly, in order not to humiliate her husband.

In the spouses' descriptions of dignity there is no doubt that both members of the couple accommodate themselves to the illness in different ways (Corbin and Strauss 1988, 6), primarily to sustain their couplehood as long as possible. Both members of the couple balance their actions in everyday life. In the example of Hans and Maria, the person with dementia actively avoids situations that could have an effect on their dignity of identity, and the cognitively intact spouse tries to maintain the involvement of the ill partner and to stress former achievements, in order not to humiliate him. Maria downplayed her husband's mistakes when he tried to do things in their home and Hans restricted his own autonomy by not going out alone. Hans, Lars, and Karl wanted to do things in the home that made them feel useful. To some extent, Hans and Karl seemed to recognize their decreased ability to perform certain tasks, in contradistinction to Lars who seemed to feel that he had a high degree of autonomy. Lisa let her husband decide more, compared to the way Maria and Eva acted, in order not to restrict Lars's feeling of autonomy. Pullman (1999, 38–39) uses the concept of *common dignity* in the context of care homes when patients have lost their capacity of autonomy. He writes that a dignity respecting paternalism is more important than an autonomy respecting paternalism. In common dignity there is a mutual interdependence between the patient and the caregiver. While respecting the basic and personal dignity of the patients, the personal dignity of the formal caregivers is enriched. In the three couples who lived with dementia a similar mutual interdependence existed. The wives seemed to balance their husband's autonomy and dignity, as well as their own, in order to sustain a feeling of being a spouse, or a care partner.

In a spousal relationship, it is the cognitively intact spouse who becomes increasingly more responsible for their common life story and their shared dignity. Lantz (2009, 170) mentions three types of storytelling: (1) first-person telling (the individual persons own narrative which defines who I am); (2) second-person telling (a narrative in dialogue); and (3) third-person telling (a narrative with an outsider perspective). All three couples had problems keeping their shared life story and the husbands with dementia had an affected ability of storytelling in all of the three types described above. Over time Hans lost his ability to speak, Lars concentrated on organizing his own life story, and Karl had forgotten parts of his own and the shared life with Eva. The biographical work is a demanding task when living with a chronic disease (Corbin and Strauss 1985, 231), a work that defines who I am and who we are as a couple.

The couple needs to accommodate not only to the dementia trajectory, but also how they as individuals are positioned by others, namely, as caretaker or caregiver instead of as a unit consisting of "two selves." None of these three couples used expressions of this kind when they narrated about their own situation in the interviews. Maria tried, very firmly, to refuse to give in to the label of caregiver. She preferred the word "support":

I support him. We have always lived together and we will continue to do that. One relative of mine said "Now when he [Hans] is ill, are you going to care for him?" But, I'll be damned. "To care for him! We are married and he is my husband!" What do they think, that you should cut the head off people or what?

In addition to avoiding the words caretaker or caregiver, none of the couples characterized the spouse with dementia as experiencing the social death that precedes the biological death (Sweeting and Gilhooly 1997, 94) and none of the cognitively intact partners described themselves as being "chained to a corpse." Indisputably there was an imbalance between the spouses, if we merely take the cognitive level into account; however, caring for another person is not exclusively dependent on cognition and recognition (Taylor 2008, 329). For example, Hans showed consideration and in a way cared for Maria by not going out on his own and waited patiently at her side when she needed to rest. It seems that the couples abstained from positioning themselves as either caretaker or caregiver. Additionally, in the case of the vulnerable dyad Lars and Lisa, they could both take the role as "giver" and "taker." O'Connor (2007, 166) argues that we should use the concept of position instead of role because of its interactional characteristics. It is too simplistic to divide two spouses with two separate roles; instead, couplehood is multidimensional, constructed and shared between the spouses.

Notes

1. John Bayley, Professor at Oxford University.
2. The trilogy consists of *Iris: A Memoir of Iris Murdoch* (1998), *Iris and the Friends: A Year of Memories* (1999), and *Widower's House* (2001).

References

Ballanger, Jesse F. 2008. "Reframing Dementia: The Policy Implications of Changing Concepts." In *Excellence in Dementia Care. Research into Practice*, edited by Murna Downs and Barbra Bowers, 492–508. Maidenhead: Open University Press.
Basting, Ann Davis. 2003. "Looking Back from Loss." *Journal of Aging Studies* 17: 87–99.
Bayley, John. 1998. *Iris. A Memoir of Iris Murdoch*. London: Abacus.
———. 1999. *Iris and the Friends: A Year of Memories*. London: Abacus.
———. 2001. *Widower's House*.
Behuniak, Susan M. 2011. "The Living Dead? The Construction of People with Alzheimer's Disease as Zombies." *Ageing & Society* 31: 70–92.
Caddel, Lisa S., and Linda Clare. 2010. "The Impact of Dementia on Self and Identity: A Systematic Review." *Clinical Psychology Review* 30: 113–126.

Corbin, Juliet M., and Anselm Strauss. 1985. "Managing Chronic Illness at Home: Three Lines of Work." *Qualitative Sociology*, 8(3): 224–247.
Corbin, Juliet M., and Anselm Strauss. 1988. *Unending Work and Care. Managing Chronic Illness at Home*. San Francisco: Jossey-Bass Publishers.
Corner, Lynne, and John Bond. 2004. "Being at Risk of Dementia: Fears and Anxieties of Older Adults." *Journal of Aging Studies* 18: 143–155.
Dunham, Charlotte C., and Julie H. Cannon. 2008. "They're Still in Control Enough to be in Control: Paradox of Power in Dementia Caregiving." *Journal of Aging Studies* 22: 45–53.
Fontana, Andrea, and Ronald W. Smith. 1989. "Alzheimer's Disease Victims: The 'Unbecoming' of Self and the Normalization of Competence." *Sociological Perspectives* 32(1): 35–46.
Hellström, Ingrid, Mike Nolan, and Ulla Lundh. 2007. "Sustaining 'Couplehood'. Spouses' Strategies for Living Positively with Dementia." *Dementia* 6(3):383–409.
Hermansson, Alice R. 1990. "Det sista året. Omsorg och vård vid livets slut [Caring in the last year of life, In Swedish]." PhD diss., Uppsala University.
Hockey, Jenny, and Allison James. 1993. *Growing Up and Growing Old*. London: Sage.
Johnstone, Megan-Jane. 2011. "Metaphors, Stigma and the 'Alzheimerization' of the Euthanasia Debate." *Dementia* 12:377–393. doi:10.1177/1471301211429168.
Kirk, Henning. 1995. "Da alderen blev en diagnose. [When old age became a diagnosis, In Danish]." PhD diss., Munksgaard: University of Copenhagen.
Lantz, Göran. 2009. "Dignity and the Dead." In *Dignity in Care for Older People*, edited by Lennart Nordenfelt, 168–189. Oxford: Wiley-Blackwell.
Leget, Carlo. 2012. "Analyzing Dignity: A Perspective from Ethics of Care." *Medicine Health Care and Philosophy* 16: 945–952. doi:10.1007/s1 1019-012-9427-3.
Macklin, Ruth. 2003. "Dignity Is a Useless Concept. It Means no More Than Respect for Persons or their Autonomy." *British Medical Journal* 327: 1419–1420.
Moody, Harry R. 1998. "Why Dignity in Old Age Matters." In *Dignity and Old Age*, edited by Robert Disch, Rose Dobrof, and Harry R. Moody, 13–38. Binghamton: The Haworth Press.
Nordenfelt, Lennart. 2009. "The Concept of Dignity." In *Dignity in Care for Older People*, edited by Lennart Nordenfelt, 26–53. Oxford: Wiley-Blackwell.
O'Connor, Deborah L. 2007. "Self-identifying as a Caregiver: Exploring the Positioning Process." *Journal of Aging Studies* 21: 165–174.
Post, Stephen G. 1995. *The Moral Challenge of Alzheimer Disease*. Baltimore, MD: The John Hopkins University Press.
Pullman, Daryl. 1999. "The Ethics of Autonomy and Dignity in Long-Term Care." *Canadian Journal on Aging* 18 (1): 26–46.
Scholl, Jane M., and Steven R. Sabat. 2008. "Stereotypes, Stereotype Threat and Ageing: Implications for the Understanding and Treatment of People with Alzheimer's Disease." *Ageing & Society* 28: 103–130.
Sweeting, Helen, and Mary Gilhooly. 1997. "Dementia and the Phenomenon of Social Death." *Sociology of Health & Illness* 19 (1): 93–117.
Taylor, Janelle S. 2008. "On Recognition, Caring, and Dementia." *Medical Anthropology Quarterly* 4 (22): 313–335.

Part Two

IDENTITY, AGENCY, AND EMBODIMENT

5

Questions of Meaning: Memory, Dementia, and the Postautobiographical Perspective

JENS BROCKMEIER

Memory enjoys a high reputation. It stands for one of most appreciated mental and public practices in Western societies. Equally a cognitive and cultural achievement and an ethical quality, memory is considered crucial not only because remembering the past—whether individual or social, personal or historical—is a virtue as such, a value in itself. It also is a foundational value for many other values: from work and everyday life to the field of history and the moral sphere. Memory is a solid ground on which to build.

The scientific study of brain and memory basks in the light of this reputation. A case in point is the cognitive neuroscience of memory. It has taken center stage far beyond the academic and clinical domains since its results apparently confirm the particular significance of its subject for the human condition. There are countless statements in the literature highlighting the importance of memory for humans' sense of self and identity, indeed, for the very idea of the human. Daniel Schacter, a leading neuroscientist, has formulated the general consensus: "Our sense of ourselves depends crucially on the subjective experience of remembering our pasts" (1996, 34). This consensus is even stronger in view of our autobiographical memories that "form the core of personal identity" (93), and this holds true, as Schacter maintains, whether or not memories take the form of narrative.

Considering this stable and wide-reaching consensus on the paramount importance of memory it is astonishing to see that there is actually little discussion about what we actually mean when we speak of "memory." Our fundamental ideas and concepts of memory are amazingly unproblematized, which is to say, they too enjoy a stable consensus and a high reputation. In this chapter I draw attention to some assumptions of our memory concepts commonly taken for granted. They are so commonsensical, I believe, because they appear stabilized and fixed through this consensus in a way that has turned "memory" into a given substantial entity, a natural kind.

These assumptions also extend to our understanding of dementia and other so-called memory disorders, especially in people suffering from Alzheimer's disease (AD). The etiological scenario follows a familiar script: the focus on dementia as a memory disorder, and on AD as an eventually fatal memory degeneration, implies that in losing their capability of autobiographical remembering, people also lose, in due and natural course, their sense of their being in time, that is, their sense of autobiographical time. Ultimately, therefore, they lose their sense of self and identity, if not their right to full personhood.

In my discussion of this scenario I critically think through how notions of autobiographical memory and time are interrelated with notions of autobiographical identity, in both the ill and the healthy. In doing so I particularly draw on recent neuroscientific findings that undergird the effort to advance an alternative view of remembering and forgetting, as well as a different, postautobiographical view of identity in persons with progressive dementia. This postautobiographical view may seem radical against the backdrop of a theoretically and culturally established (and normatively sanctioned) conception of memory; yet it is not such a far-fetched idea for many clinical practitioners and caretakers, as we will see in the last section of the chapter. To give an idea of the problem at stake I start out with sketching three characters and three different scenes illustrating different aspects of the issue I want to examine.

Iris Murdoch, the Memory Killer, John Locke

The first character is Iris Murdoch, the Irish-born British writer and philosopher. The scene is a television event in the 1990s that became iconic because in this show Murdoch, a shrewd public intellectual, acted in a way that made it clear to a large audience that she obviously was suffering from some kind of dementia—which, in fact, later turned out to be the onset of AD. Murdoch first believed her trouble remembering and concentrating was an expression of writer's block. This perception is still evident in the television scene and in other situations described by her husband and later biographer John Bayley (1999). In one such situation, she failed to remember the name of the British Prime Minister. As she put it, "The name of the Prime Minister? I don't know, but I'm sure someone does."

There are countless situations in which a particular name or some specific bit of knowledge is actually quite irrelevant for a conversation, as was the Prime Minister's name in Murdoch's emblematic scene. Nevertheless, the question that popped up for many viewers of that television program was, Isn't it Alzheimer's? The question implies a conclusion that is almost intuitively drawn if people witness something like Murdoch's failing in what is considered to be one of memory's crucial functions: remembering important names like those of one's spouse or children or, as in this case, that of the British Prime Minister. One might object that the assumption that remembering the names of people equals remembering the people themselves is strange on its own; still, it is commonly taken to be an early indicator of AD and other dementias. In later stages, persons with memory problems are diagnosed as being disoriented in time (not knowing the day of the week, day of the month, or year), in place (not knowing where they are, where they were born, and where they live), and in person (not knowing who they or others around them are). All these forms reflect what in a different vocabulary is called problems of semantic memory. In fact, everyone who has experience with individuals with dementia has stories to tell about how they are confused and disoriented about these aspects of their existence. Yet there is more to it than the difficulty of remembering "objective" knowledge. Individuals are viewed as confused and disoriented first of all because they cannot remember pieces or even complex aspects of knowledge considered essential to one's identity and to living a life. Memory failures in respect of person or person names, place, and time thus are considered to be crucial features of the subjective and intersubjective experience of dementia. They work as intuitive indicators.

The research literature qualifies these intuitive indicators by pointing out that memory problems are the most frequent complaints of sufferers from dementia, as well as of people who live with and care for them. A second reason for the focus on memory becomes obvious if we consider its prominence in scientific studies on and in medical diagnostics of dementia. Besides disorientation, the core criterion for the standard neurological, psychiatric, and neuropsychological diagnosis of AD is "early significant episodic memory impairment, with objective evidence on testing"[1] Accordingly, memory and dementia are defined in view of what is testable, with tests designed to distinguish three forms of memory: (1) episodic cued memory, (2) episodic free memory, and (3) episodic semantic memory. These standardized memory tests—all based on measuring responses to different kinds of controlled cueing—are understood as establishing "the core amnestic deficit of AD," with the underlying assumption that "episodic-cued and episodic-semantic factor scores achieve[d] the highest accuracy in predicting AD" (Jacova 2009, 99).

A third reason for the central role memory and memory failure play in our understanding of dementia is their prominence in countless everyday accounts, fictional and nonfictional, and autobiographical and biographical representations in all kinds of media formats. Kurt Danziger (2008) pointed out that modern Western cultures have developed an obsession with memory, and that is with a particular idea of memory, namely, with memory as a quantifiable, testable, verifiable, and reliable entity, an information storage. This view also has shaped the perception (and definition) of memory failures and disorders. Against this background, equally manifest in clinical, academic, and common sense discourses, AD first and foremost has become a memory disease—a "memory killer," as we can read in popular publications.

Interestingly, despite the heterogeneity of these three kinds of discourse on memory and dementia there is astonishing agreement on what memory *is*. Memory, as already mentioned, is conceived of a physiologically localizable capacity, structure, or property of the brain—or, more precisely, as "a collection of mental abilities that use different systems and components within the brain to retain information over time" (Budson, 2011), to quote just one definition out of an extended but homonymous literature of clinical and neuroscientific textbooks, research reports, and self-help publications. On this account, memory is understood after the model of an organ, or a part of an organ, that can be affected by various dementias, such as AD, the "memory killer," just like the lung can be affected by cancer. The memory killer is typically identified in terms of senile plaque or tangles that, like germs, bacteria, or fungus, aggressively attack what is most valuable to us. The memory killer fits well Susan Sontag's (1978) description of illness metaphors that suggest an external enemy attacking a person or their body, an attack against which the person has to fight back. If this fight cannot be won, the affected part of someone's body or mind has to be given up or replaced like a hip, heart, or lung.

The problem with dementia, however, is that this metaphorical formula does not work; nor does it work with other so-called memory disorders. One reason is that neither memory nor memory disorders can be localized as a well-defined and marked-off entity (or capability, or structure, or system, or network of systems) in the same way as, say, an anatomist can do it with a lung, and sometimes even with the cancerous parts of it. Nor are we able to adequately assess, much less quantitatively measure, the "performance" of memory through neuropsychological tests. Harking back to William Stern's (1921) critique of diagnostic tests as providing only an unreliable "momentary snapshot of the performance capabilities of the examinee," Steven Sabat (2001; 2013) has argued that neuropsychological test profiles are created under artificial conditions that do not have much in common with people's agentive nature and their actual abilities to interact, think, and plan. They often focus on recalling information that is isolated, taken out of the context of everyday social life, and clinically individualized. Moreover, being confronted with a clinical testing situation whose outcome can have existential consequences is, for many people, downright anxiety provoking. Since anxiety, as is well known, can essentially diminish cognitive (including mnemonic) performances—in fact, it can disorient people, and not only those who are threatened with being diagnosed as victims of the "memory killer"—test results appear even more insignificant. What is more, diagnostic tests exclude narrative capabilities, that is, precisely those capabilities that afford most individuals the most natural (and, at the same time, most complex) way to deal with existential challenges. This is all the more important because even people in the moderate or severe stages of dementia are able, at least to some degree, to tell stories about themselves and their world (Hydén 2013; Usita, Hyman, and Herman 1998; 2006). Narrative creates a unique experiential and communicative space that proves to be particularly helpful under such extreme circumstances (Medved and Brockmeier 2008).

These arguments resonate with an alternative tradition of neuroscientific and biomedical voices. A number of scientists in this tradition off the beaten track believe that it is impossible to understand how the brain works if it is reduced to an isolated and self-contained entity viewed in isolation from the person whose organ it is and from the social and cultural life of this person (see, Gazzaniga 2006; Rose 2006; Singer 2006; 2008). This tradition can be viewed as building on earlier work by Kurt Goldstein (1934/1995) and Alexander Luria (1973), among others. It has also been elaborated by philosophers of mind (e.g., Noë 2009; Clark 2011), psychologists (e.g., Gergen 2010), and anthropologists (e.g. Ingold 2012). One essential point of this tradition is captured by Ingold's formulation that, ultimately, the brain is social because life is social. That brains are in the service of the person and his or her social life is attended by an important differentiation: brains work according to physiological laws and causal necessities, whereas persons are agents who act intentionally and intersubjectively according to social requirements and culturally developed meanings and values. In other words, persons act on reasons, not only causes (Brockmeier 1996).

Furthermore, persons are able to reflect on their actions and on themselves, taking on individual responsibility according to such social requirements and cultural values. This implies that it is people, not brains, who think, believe, evaluate, and take decisions—even if many neuroscientists attribute such intentional and reflexive states to neurological processes and systems, "ascribing psychological predicates" to a material "Inner Entity," as Bennett and Hacker (2003, 81) put it. There are of course individual differences and degrees of constriction and limitations in respect of agency and intentionality, but this does not detract from the principle at stake. It is a principle that holds for all human beings whether they are challenged by diseases (e.g., AD), injuries (e.g., neurotrauma), syndromes (e.g., autism), or (genetic) neurological disabilities (Medved and Brockmeier 2010).

In contrast with this picture, traditional clinical and neuroscientific memory tests put forward an idea of memory as a well-defined and marked-off physical entity or system, a natural kind whose capacities can be isolated and measured. The design and theoretical framework of standard diagnostic tests build on the established psychological and neuroscientific model of memory as storage—a system or a set of systems that encodes, stores, and retrieves knowledge or information from the past. This knowledge concerns various domains, one of which is autobiographical. Autobiographical knowledge results from a person's own experience, specifically from experience that is linked to one's self in time (or one's identity).

Why does this model presume such a close connection between identity and time, that is, a specific concept of time? At the heart of this connection is the idea of personal identity as bound to the temporal trajectory of one's autobiographical past, present, and future. In the neuroscientific age, this trajectory is viewed as a biologically anchored sense of time, we might even say, as remembered time. This sense permits us, via remembering and prediction (or "foresight"), to localize our experiences and thus ourselves as beings that are continuous in time. Creating a temporally ordered chain of episodic memories, we are able to time travel backward and forward, reminiscing past and predicting future events (Bar 2011; Suddendorf and Corballis 2007).

On this view, structuring our lives chronologically, from the beginning to the end, is the natural mode of becoming aware of our autobiographical time. It is this "chronological sense" of one's being in time that is fundamental not only for one's chronological time consciousness, but also for the emergence of one's sense of being a person and having an identity, since both are essentially defined as continuous. Considering this conception as a whole, it makes sense that it is closely associated with the dominant idea of memory that I have already outlined from various points of view, the idea of memory as an archive that permits us to recall the past in a chronological order and, in the light of this past, assess the present and anticipate the future. This is the standard view of memory, identity, and autobiographical time, the neuroscientific and clinical paradigm for assessing the healthy and diagnosing the sick.

As comprehensive and well-founded as this view may appear—a case in point are the twenty-five chapters in Bar (2011), many of which are authored by leading researchers in the field—there is a lot it does not capture. To begin with the point just mentioned, postulating a naturally chronological sense of one's lifetime imposes an abstract Newtonian model of time on human brains and minds that leaves out of account the large individual and cultural variety in how we understand and live with time, including autobiographical time (Brockmeier 2000; 2009). In addition, a basic feature of this view is to exclude conceiving of personhood, identity, and autobiographical time in a contextualized way, in a way that localizes processes of remembering not only in the brain, but also in the social and embedded practices of persons, in their cultural forms of life. It thus rules out a view of identity or sense of self that is less, or possibly not at all, grounded in autobiographical memory but in forms of action and interaction. These social and cultural forms of life are constitutive of our being in the world. They range from practices of self-localization in narrative and other discursive ways of self-resolution to embodied, intersubjective, and performative practices of self-experience and communication. Differently put, the standard view ignores any idea of identity or sense of self that does *not* center on the assumption of its anchorage in autobiographical memory, on a notion of personal identity as autobiographical identity.

Be it despite or because of this restriction, there can be little doubt that the standard notion has dominated Western conceptions of self and personal identity in an amazingly persistent tradition since John Locke. Locke, the eighteen-century English philosopher and physician, can be said to be the father of the orthodoxy that personal identity is autobiographical, that there is only one continuity that allows for the claim of individual identity: the continuity of autobiographical memories that are represented in one's consciousness. Locke's (2008/1690) theory of mind is the first conception of the self as grounded in the continuity of one's consciousness in time. It postulates that humans have no other way to establish their identity as persons than by their individual memories of themselves. The identity of a person, Locke maintained, depends on their existence as "a thinking, intelligent being, that has reason and reflection, and can consider itself as itself, the same thinking thing, in different times and places" (II, Chap. 27, 9.). As this apparently has been such a convincing, in fact, taken-for-granted idea both in everyday thinking and in philosophical reflection about issues of identity and dementia (Matthews 2006), it is not surprising that it also underlies the neuroscientific and clinical vision of memory and identity in dementia research and diagnostics. It thus even undergirds the perception of AD as "the memory killer," giving theoretical support to the disregard of other ways of understanding human identity and memory, under both conditions of health and illness— ways that are discussed in the chapters of this book.

What is the Reality of Concepts?

To be sure it was not the thought of an individual seventeenth-century philosopher but an array of historical and cultural circumstances and factors that has made the Lockean model of memory and identity so pervasive. Still, we deal with a conceptual model, so let me dwell for a moment on the question of what kind of conceptual entities we are talking about when we talk about "identity," "memory," and "time." To what do these terms refer? What is their mode of being, their ontology?

When we find these concepts used in discourses about AD and other forms of dementia their ontology is commonly straightforward: they refer to natural kinds, that is, they purport to represent properties and qualities of the given, material world. Once they are considered natural kinds with the same ontological status, it seems relatively easy to examine correlations between these entities. We can see this in much of the experimental research on the relationship between autobiographical memory and identity in individuals with AD. A not unusual example is a study by Addis and Tippett (2004) that employs a wide spectrum of test batteries for measuring memory and identity, both modeled as exclusively inner-individual constructs of quantifiable variables. At the same time, however, a crucial function of these test designs is to construe exactly the well-defined memory ontology they pretend to assess. As a consequence, in such studies the focus on method—or perhaps better, on experimental and measurement techniques—overrides all other aspects (Caddell and Clare 2010). In line with this orientation the main interest is in the correlation of autobiographical memory and identity in AD as such, that is in the disease as a self-contained entity, rather than in persons who are struggling with it in an individual and highly personal way. Not surprisingly, the result of the study just mentioned is the generic and universal finding "that autobiographical memory loss affects identity" (Addis and Tippett 2004, 56), among others, by lessening its "strength" and "quality."

The notion of memory has always been the subject of strong substantialist and naturalist attributions. Today there seems to be a near-consensus among scientific memory researchers that what they investigate is a natural kind, a part or property of the material world (Danziger 2008; Hacking 1996; Michaelian 2010). However, there also have been strong counterarguments drawing on different traditions of thought. These traditions view what is meant by the noun "memory" less as an individual capacity or system and more as a process or a plethora of societally, culturally, and historically embedded processes of remembering and forgetting. The claim here is that the concept of memory belongs to the same family of concepts as "identity" and "person." These concepts do not denote given objects of the material world but rather indicate unstable meaning constructions ascribed to and negotiated among individuals who, in the process, are defined and redefined by others and by themselves. Qualified from different points of view and in different vocabularies, this definition has been called transactional (Bruner 1987), discursive (Harré and Gillett 1994), performative (Butler 1990), epistemic (Foucault 1970), and narrative (Bruner 1990; Ricoeur 1992; Lindemann Nelson 2001), among others. One important feature these definitions share is that they represent not only a conceptual or otherwise discursive and narrative effect but try to capture this effect as intertwined with real actions. In this way, identity appears to be realized in the process in which people act out their personhood: it is not so much expressed in actions (including discursive and narrative actions) as created by being enacted or, as Butler put it, "performatively constituted by the very 'expressions' that are said to be its result" (1990, 25).

An implication of this argument is that these performative expressions are locally and historically variable cultural practices. They are part and parcel of both everyday discourses and of the special reflective and conceptual efforts to understand them, such as the scientific and theoretical endeavors of neuroscientists, psychologists, philosophers, and social scientists. Whatever the concepts of identity and person used in these discourses refer to, they cannot be envisioned, let alone understood, without taking into account the social and cultural dynamics in which they are brought up—which means, in which they are interpreted, negotiated, and contested. This applies to both kinds of discourses, to those at home in everyday life (with its manifold performative modes from the embodied to the symbolically mediated), and to those in the reflexive, scientific-theoretical domain (with its various institutional orders and conceptions of evidence and plausibility). By the same token it is irrelevant whether the study of the cultural reality of personhood concentrates on experience-based concepts of identity from the former kind of discourse (sometimes called *emic* concepts), or on analytical and investigative concepts (sometimes called *etic*) from the latter kind.

Essential, on this account, for the understanding of what identity means and what it refers to is the role of symbolic, communicative, and, especially, linguistic forms of action and interaction. One prominent example of such a form and practice is narrative. Narrative plays a crucial role in our understanding of human identity, and it does so both on an emic, everyday experience-based level and on an etic, theoretical and conceptual level (Brockmeier 2012). What makes it such an important practice is, not least, its intimate intermingling with other contextual and embodied practices of communication and self-resolution, to the degree that these practices can realize important aspects of narrative discourse even without the use of words and other speech elements. Both its "embedded quality" (Georgakopoulou 2007; Herman 2011) and its "embodied quality" (Hydén 2013; Kontos 2004) make narrative a particularly important practice of interaction and self-reassurance for individuals with dementia or aphasia.

This cultural and performative conception of the person and his or her identity is well known in the social sciences and the humanities. However, this cannot be said about the understanding of memory, which is widely regarded as physical or biological given, as natural kind. In this respect, the research fields of neuroscience, clinical-biomedical studies, and social sciences are in accordance; and this also comprises those quarters of the social sciences and humanities that otherwise are inclined to discursive, social-constructivist, and cultural approaches. This is not the place to explore the complex reasons for this almost commonsensical agreement on a biologically given ontology of individual memory—its status as a natural kind—which is epistemologically remarkable enough. What I want to do is to make the same case for memory that I just laid out for identity.

I therefore zoom in on memory's temporal dimension that, as we remember, often figures as a central diagnostic criterion for dementia. But before that let me add a word about my work—studying practices of remembering and forgetting as well as "memory discourses" in various cultural contexts. Patent in these contexts are some fundamental changes in the understanding of memory and autobiographical memory, in particular, which have occurred over the last decades in a number of areas of research often independent from the biologically and cognitively oriented mainstream of experimental memory study (Brockmeier 2010). It is on the observation of these changes that I want to base my case. In a nutshell, there are many findings suggesting that the idea of memory as we have long known and appreciated it in the West is in the midst of a crisis. Part of this crisis is that the conception of memory as an archive—to be described and imagined in terms of encoding, storing, and recalling of information—is dissolving. Instead, new perspectives have gained importance that foreground a broad variety of practices and artifacts of remembering and forgetting that reach far beyond the individual domain of consciousness (including the unconscious), cognition, and neurocognition, a domain that so far has been conceptualized as a kind of neurobiological storehouse of the past.

What is changing here is not just some detail in our knowledge of memory but rather memory's historical ontology. Historical ontology is a term proposed by Ian Hacking (1995; 2002) to describe the interplay between the notion of memory and what is taken to be its material reality. I have already used the concept ontology to refer to the particular status or kind of being that we ascribe to a phenomenon or a class of phenomena. What does it mean to see memory's ontology as historical? In Hacking's analysis, the ontology of memory is not that of a universal biological entity but something that came into being as an epistemic subject in the wake of the emerging memory sciences in the nineteenth century. The new "scientific approach" to memory extended to three fields that were only casually connected: (1) the neurological study of different "types" of memory; (2) the experimental studies of recall; and (3) the clinical, psychoanalytical, or psychodynamic studies of memory. In the twentieth century, these fields were joined by biological research on the cell level and computer modeling or cognitive science. Hacking (1995) shows that this originally late nineteenth-century movement set out to transform what was until then called the "soul" into a subject of positive natural-science investigation. Driving this point further, I argue that now, little more than a century later, the same epistemic subject "memory" is about to dissolve, and that this dissolution comes in tandem with a number of new scientific, technological, and cultural developments that override the old archival idea of memory.

The upshot of Hacking's (1995) inquiry is that memory is one of those epistemic entities that not only represent and define, but also structure, evoke, and to a certain degree constitute the reality to which they refer. On this view, there are various interactions between concepts and the "reality" of the entities to which they refer. These interactions are different in diverse concept-reality relationships. It would be preposterous, Hacking maintains, to believe that the only thing material objects, such as planets, have in common is that we call them planets. The similarities and differences of sun, moon, and the celestial bodies called planets are real enough; they are not just a consequence of our concepts. There are, however, things that differ from planets and the like, as there are different categories, and these are closer to our concerns here. These categories do not refer in such a straightforward manner to phenomena of nature, such as celestial bodies. Take gloves as an example. The concept of glove, Hacking argues, fits gloves so well because we made them that way (2002, 106–107). We might view human beings or persons, and what we call their identities and memories, in a similar fashion. In a few important respects persons are more like gloves than like planets; even here the category and the people it refers to emerged hand in hand. Hacking calls this a mutual process of "making up people," a process that involves an interplay between human beings and the historical category of a person as a politically, legally, philosophically, and psychologically defined modern individual.

In much of the prototypical natural sciences our categories do not really change the way the world works. However, the matter is different when it comes to human beings and parts or aspects of them, such as identity and memory. Prototypical human sciences are characterized by a continuous dialogue between concepts and systems of description and classification and the people they categorize and classify. This is particularly important, not least in political respects, in disciplines that examine aspects of people and their lives in terms of psychic or mental diseases, such as trauma, hysteria, schizophrenia, obsessive-compulsive disorder, or multiple personality disorder. Here the dialogue is all but symmetrical. In all of these fields there are definitions of human "normalcy" that also regard "healthy" and "normal" or otherwise normative forms and practices of remembering and forgetting; on some of these I have already touched. With this excursion in mind, I want to consider few of the changes in our understanding of memory.

Dissolving the Archive of Memory

According to the Lockean view an essential function of human consciousness is to keep us on track of the chronological order of "our" time, our autobiographical time. It is the chain of autobiographical memories that allows us to become aware of our being in time in terms of past, present, and future. This view has essentially contributed not only to the conceptual shape of the modern idea of memory but also to our clinical and diagnostic approaches to dementia. Beyond the biomedical and clinical sphere, it also dominates public discourses on dementia. However, as I have emphasized, neither our conceptions of memory and dementia, nor of identity and time can be understood outside of the interplay between concept and reality just outlined. In fact, what has been called the recent "memory crisis" entails that this interplay has become particularly active with respect to these concepts.

Although the tendency of questioning the idea of human memory as a device for storing and later retrieval of experiences can also be observed in the fields of biomedical and neurocognitive research, it has only to a very limited degree affected the very conceptual layout of memory in this domain. In all psychological and neuroscientific standard textbooks and reference works on memory and learning that I have reviewed, the focus on brain mechanisms of remembering and forgetting and its conceptualization in terms of encoding, storing or retaining, and retrieval of information remains unchanged. The continuity of this conceptual tradition is all the more astonishing because many new findings and observations in this research domain challenge the archival model of memory. Is there a new generation of researchers about to replace the last generation of researchers (and textbook authors) who still spent most of their academic life under the hegemony of traditional cognitive models that seem to have seamlessly migrated into the new age of brain science, but now reach their limits? A brief review of some of the novel findings may give a sense of where these new trends are headed. I limit myself to three.

REMEMBERING AND PERCEIVING

I start with a few new insights of brain research that have a direct bearing on our construction of "the past."[2] Storing and recalling past experience is, according to the traditional doctrine, the common denominator of what memory is all about. Now considering matters on neurocognitive and neurobiological levels, one of the most bewildering new findings is that there is no evident distinction between brain processes operative in remembering and in perceiving. We also could say that there is no biological correlate that allows us to distinguish between what we traditionally call acts of remembering the past from acts of perceiving the present. And this is true for the visual, acoustical, and tactile mode. Nor are there any indicators that separate the content of a perception in the here and now from the content of one that we had at some point in the past. For the neuronal circuits involved, there is no difference between perceiving a person here and now and having perceived this person a few days or years ago. This raises the question, If it is not a neurobiological configuration, what then makes us discriminate between the present of a perception and the past of a memory? It is we who attribute it afterward in an act of interpretation and temporal localization. This act is one of creation, not just of representation or mirroring; it integrates a number of activities on the levels of the brain, the mind, and the culture in which both the mind and the brain are embedded.

PERCEIVING AND IMAGINING

Other studies report that the same applies for the distinction between a present perception or thought and an imagined future perception or thought, a distinction that likewise is unverifiable on neurological grounds. Whether I perceive a person or imagine the person (regardless of whether I want to or am afraid to meet or perceive this person in the future), the activated neuronal functions are the same. Several neuroscientists have demonstrated that the brain abilities involved when I recall a scene at the last Thanksgiving dinner (an "episodic memory") and when I imagine this scene to happen at a future Thanksgiving dinner (a "episodic future thought" or "foresight") are indistinguishable. This is confirmed by research on patients with amnesia who find it equally hard to imagine new experiences and conjure up holistic scenarios in the future.[3]

REAL AND IMAGINED EMOTIONS

Within the same field of research, it has been shown that feelings associated with perceptions make use of the same neuronal processes as feelings associated with imaginings. Identical neuronal activities are involved in my emotional reaction to a person I see in the present, to the memory of that person (be it mental or mediated through a photograph), or to an imagined future encounter with that person. Again, the same imaginative capacities and emotional states are active when people have certain thoughts, beliefs, or desires, or imagine having these thoughts, beliefs, or desires at whatever point in time. All studies in this area suggest that there is no such thing as a physiological borderline between what we consider and "feel" to be present (that is, what we perceive or experience in the here and now), future (what we anticipate in our imagination), and past (what we usually call memory). Once more the question arises, What then defines a "memory" if it is not given, identifiable, or deducible through a neurophysiological substrate in the brain? How do we qualify an experience as past experience, as a memory?

Time and Temporalization

This question brings into view the temporal status of an experience—and thus another question: how do we gauge this status? Many of our experiences are temporally localized; we take them, for example, as something that occurs presently or belongs to the past or the future. Moreover, we view them as something that happens simultaneously, earlier, or later in relation to other experiences. These are the two basic ways in which we order events "in time," or, as we also might call it, we temporalize them. I prefer to put it the latter way because, within the framework I have suggested, this is not to say that these forms of temporalization necessarily reflect a given natural kind, an ontological property of the world in which we live. Nor can this or any other notion of time be said to reflect the reality or nature of a physical or neurobiological time trajectory that preexists our concepts of it, as though it were independent of the meaning constructions by which we strive to temporalize our experiences.

If, instead, we view chronological time in the wake of Einstein as a model by which we think and organize our experiences, not as a given condition under which we live, then we can find abundant confirmation in the recent neurobiological studies presented above because all of them tend to desubstantialize our sense of time. Looking at the matter from this point of view shifts attention from the question of how we autobiographically localize ourselves "in time," which is what many neuropsychological memory tests try to measure, to something else, namely, to how we localize ourselves in meaningful contexts by—possibly—using temporal assumptions and constructions, which is beyond the reach of any of these tests.

I do not claim that the two ways of temporalization just delineated are our only ways. Irrespective of how many different ways there are in which we temporalize our experiences and ourselves, the point I want to make is that they are to be conceived of as ways of action, as forms of life. Our strategies of temporalization encompass a large variety of meaning-making activities; and they include activities of consciousness that are more comprehensive than those realized exclusively on a neurobiological level, which is not to say that this is not complex enough already. Yet the complexity at stake also spans the societal and cultural dimension of human consciousness, and so it also comprises consciousness' interlacement with sign and symbol systems, such as language.

Our conscious temporal experience is not just sequential and homogeneous, nor is it primarily shaped by chronological time orders, such as the hour, the month, and the year. Rather, our experiences are temporalized by the meanings that we give them and through which we perceive of and reflect on them. These meanings are inextricably intermingled with our life worlds, with passions, beliefs, and idiosyncratic concerns. Because these forms of life do not show up on the radar of neuropsychological tests or assessments of dementia, they necessitate more embedded and contextualized hermeneutic approaches. These approaches have to be sensitive to particular subjectivities and ways of identity; this includes the ways of people whose autobiographical memories and times may only play a peripheral role for their sense of self and identity.

Against this backdrop it is instructive to consider some further findings from neuroscientific research, neuropathological studies, and other clinical observations suggesting a direct link between the *imaginative* trajectories of memory and time. Because we cannot on neuronal grounds distinguish the perception of a person from the imagination of this person—whether we set the imagined person in the past or future—we cannot separate "real" acts of remembering from acts of "imagined" or "simulated" remembering. What characterizes the mental simulation of either factual or hypothetical scenarios is that it draws on a mix of experience and fictitious imagination, and that this mix makes use of the same constructive brain activities (Hassabis and Maguire 2007, 299). Some scientists dub what happens in these processes "mental scene construction" or "self-projection," or they refer to the creative "navigating" of a "prospective brain" (see chapters in Bar, 2011).

Consider a constellation in which we have trouble remembering the guests at a birthday party we attended a few weeks ago. What we typically do is to compel our brains to imagine what it would be like if we were about to sit at the same dinner table again. Where, then, would one draw the line between imagination and recollection? Just as it has always been questionable to draw such a borderline on psychological grounds, so now we know that it is impossible on neurobiological grounds. As Edelman (2006) writes, the very complexity of describing a remembering brain arises from the fact that "every act of perception is to some degree an act of creation, and every act of memory is to same degree an act of imagination" (100).

Decentering Memory and the Postautobiographical View

There are different ways to gain insights and create new knowledge. One is to analyze empirical phenomena, another is to examine the concepts, models, and theories through which these empirical phenomena are identified, classified, and understood. Sometimes these two go hand in hand, as in Hacking's example of the glove and the concept of the glove. If you have a model of memory, the empirical phenomena are observed and "the data" collected in a way that is likely to confirm the model and the underlying theory. The model examined in this chapter draws on the traditional conception of memory as a storage of the past, which comes in tandem with the neurobiologically grounded idea of autobiographical identity—personal identity that is based on autobiographical memory. For a long time, this model has provided the neuroscientific underpinning of a picture of dementia ubiquitous in neuropsychological and clinical literature and practice. In taking a closer look at recent changes in our understanding of memory, I have foregrounded the radical challenges for the traditional model of memory that these changes entail. At the center of my discussion has been the interplay between the concept and the reality of this construct, a discussion which has emphasized that the ontology claimed by traditional notions of autobiographical memory and autobiographical time is all but stable and empirically given. Building on an argument by Hacking I have proposed this ontology as a set of historical and cultural assumptions that presently are once again in the midst of a far-ranging transformation.

Against this background, one of the views I have questioned is that dementia is linked to the pathological degeneration or dissolution of a supposedly natural sense of chronological time. There are some much-discussed examples of such putative linkage in the neurosciences, such as Tulving's (2002) idea of "chronesthesia," or conceptions of remembering and foresight as forms of mental time travel (Suddendorf and Corballis 2007; Suddendorf, Addis, and Corballis 2011). Common to these studies—and echoed in the clinical literature—is the presupposition that there is an intimate connection between a person's autobiographical remembering and his or her sense of time; the implication is that both are essential for the formation of identity because identity is based on the temporal chain of one's autobiographical memories. Once these assumptions are accepted, a close correlation between neurodegenerative memory problems and personal identity suggests itself. If, instead, we take the view that there is no reason to assume the existence of a biological substrate that immediately corresponds to, or even determines, our practices of remembering and our sense of time—as much as there is no reason to assume such a substrate to our constructions of identity—then identity, memory, and autobiographical time equally appear as meaning formations.

Of course this is not to deny the reality of amyloid plaques and tangles, the celestial bodies of dementia research, and the necessity to investigate their impact on the brain. But it is to argue that there is no direct and causal way from neurotransmitters and the neurodegeneration that prevents them from transmitting properly to the intersubjective and cultural constructions of autobiographical identity, memory, and time. It is in this light that many standard definitions of dementia as well as clinical test and assessment instruments need to be critically scrutinized. A further consequence of this view is that it requires us to explore the full range of actions and interactions through which individuals localize themselves in terms of identity and personhood, rather than just narrowing down this exploration to acts of autobiographical remembering that the Lockean model claimed to be essential for one's sense of temporal continuity and identity.

I think, for example, of ethnographic, phenomenological, and clinical work—some of which is presented in this volume—that investigates intersubjective practices of self-localization, such as narrative and other embodied activities of persons with dementia. Such activities are much more meaningful, agentive, and intelligible manifestations of identity and self than the decontextualized skills measured in neurocognitive memory tests can possibly capture. All too often the focus on the general *mechanics* of memory tends to neglect paying heed to the particular *meanings* memories might possess for individuals, as William Randall (2011, 22) puts it. Not surprisingly, interest in approaches to dementia that go beyond the focus on neurodegeneration and declining memory and its impact on identity is more likely to be found among clinicians and caretakers—one example is the work of Tom Kitwood (1997)—than among scientists and diagnosticians.

I want to end by pointing to two further examples of the work of these clinicians and practitioners. One is the Trebus Project. The United Kingdom–based project is a memory archive that collects the narratives of people with dementia in various media, placing particular emphasis on what the storytellers have to say about their experience of dementia and the problems it has caused (The Trebus Project 2012). Drawing on many years of experience in working with affected individuals, David Clegg, one of the project's protagonists, reports that memory problems and the lack of autobiographical memories, in particular, are not at the heart of most people's concerns.

> Although many people progress through the stages of a dementia with surprising calmness, resilience and humor, some do not. Spending over 6,000 hours in one-to-one sessions with people with dementia…has convinced me that the greatest difficulty for some may not be what they forget at the beginning of their dementia so much as the feeling of loss, the petty conflicts, the lost hopes, the family disputes, the anxieties and financial hardships, that they cannot resolve, come to terms with, or stop themselves remembering at the end. (Clegg 2010)

The ways in which neuropsychological tests and diagnostic instruments to assess memory performances are failing to capture the complex psychological reality of lives and minds has also been described by Anne Basting (2009). Inspired and motivated by her background in theater, Basting is one of a growing number of clinical practitioners in North America who have been developing ways to embed creative and artistic practices into long-term care. This seems astonishing in the light of traditional perceptions of persons with dementia that claim a general decline of cognitive abilities, and surely of creative ones. But as these perceptions change, there is a shift in focus of attention from individual cognitive capacities like memory to social forms of life that are embedded, embodied, and enacted. Basting has made plain how she was disappointed and frustrated with the failure of reminiscing techniques and memory training programs. When she finally gave up on them she started experimenting with new creative activity and interaction formats that ignore any special attention to memory performances. Why, she wondered, would long-term care exclude free storytelling in groups, playwriting, acting, and other social practices of imagination?

> When people hear the word "dementia," they think decline and loss. They don't tend to think of growth. I …have been…trying to teach people that growth and loss aren't mutually exclusive. Dementia certainly entails some loss of ability with language, even in the early stage, but there are so many other ways to express one's self. Creativity and the arts can open up a whole new world to people with a progressive memory disorder. They offer a way to make meaning, leave legacy, and connect with friends, care partners, and future generations. (Basting 2009/10)

Projects and experiences like Clegg's and Basting's reflect various aspects of what it means to decenter memory or, at least, to decenter the traditional understanding of autobiographical memory that I have discussed in this chapter. They suggest that such decentering brings to the fore a new, wider, postautobiographical view of identity. This view may also permit us to get a better sense of the peculiar "dilemmas of being" that increasingly define living a life with dementia, as Mark Freeman (2008) has described it in observing his mother struggling with AD. For a long while, she appeared to be quite aware of many of the complications this life entails, first of all caused by her poor memory. Often, Freeman remarks, she is tired and frustrated, exhausted from all the trouble and discomfort of her situation, feeling at times that her autobiographical self and the many narratives that constitute it are about to disappear. She even is aware of the threatening consequences of this disappearance. However, there also is a reluctance to accept this, an unwillingness to give in and succumb to what this impressive woman seems to perceive as a great injustice being done to her. In doing so, "she remains committed," Freeman writes, "strenuously, to pressing on, being her own person, keeping herself as connected to the world as possible" (2008, 178). In this sense, there seems to be a "sense of sameness," as ephemeral as it may be, a feeling of "continuity in discontinuity," of being someone who has a sense of oneself even without remembering the autobiographical whereabouts, as Freeman notes on his mother in another work (2010, 173). What appears to make itself felt here is the desire of world-connectedness and self-connectedness in an "'I' who reflects upon the 'me' that has emerged only to find its radical difference and otherness" (2010, 173).

What I have called the postautobiographical view encourages us not only to realize such "dilemmas of being"—the deeply rooted will and desire to keep oneself "as connected to the world as possible" even and particularly when facing a development that centrally aims at dissolving this connection. It also affords us to bear in mind what a multitude of such connections there is, a multitude that essentially contributes to one's sense of self and identity, and that many of these connections are independent from any autobiographical mooring in one's past. The postautobiographical view of identity goes beyond the fixation on the proper mnemonic storage and retrieval of one's past; it goes beyond the fixation on one's past at all. In defying the Lockean imperative of autobiographical memory, it opens up novel perspectives on the multiple forms and practices in and through which humans enact their identities.

Notes

1. See for example Jacova (2009); Jacova et al. (2007); Dubois et al. (2007).
2. The neuroscientific research dealing with this issue is extensive. In the following summaries I draw especially on Addis, Wong, and Schacter (2007); Addis et al. (2009); Bar (2011); Gazzaniga, Ivry, and Mangum (2009); Edelman (2006); Nelson (2007); Schacter (1996; 2002); Schacter, Addis, and Buckner (2008); Spreng, Mar, and Kim (2009); Suddendorf and Corballis (2007); Suddendorf, Addis, and Corballis (2011); Szpunar (2010); Szpunar, Watson, and McDermott (2007); Szpunar, Chan, and McDermott (2009); Szpunar and Tulving (2011); if not otherwise referenced.
3. See Hassabis et al. (2007); Klein, Loftus, and Kihlstrom (2002).

References

Addis, Donna R., and Lynette Tippett. 2004. "Memory of Myself: Autobiographical Memory and Identity in Alzheimer's Disease." *Memory* 12: 56–74.

———, L. Pan, M. A. Vu, N. Laiser, and Daniel Schacter. 2009. "Constructive Episodic Simulation of the Future and the Past: Distinct Subsystems of a Core Brain Network Mediate Imagining and Remembering." *Neuropsychologia* 47: 2222–2238.

———, A. T. Wong, and Daniel Schacter. 2007. "Remembering the Past and Imagining the Future: Common and Distinct Neuronal Substrates during Event Construction and Elaboration." *Neuropsychologia* 45: 1363–1377.

Bar, Moshe, ed. 2011. *Predictions in the Brain: Using our Past to Generate a Future*. New York & Oxford: Oxford University Press.

Basting, Anne. 2009. *Forget Memory: Creating Better Lives for People with Dementia*. Baltimore, MD: Johns Hopkins University Press.

———. 2009/10. Five Questions for Anne Basting. The Alzheimer's Association, New York Chapter. Accessed 21 January 2014 http://www.alznyc.org/newsletter/spring2008/06.asp

Bayley, John. 1999. *Elegy for Iris*. New York: St. Martin's Press

Bennett, Maxwell, and Peter M. S. Hacker. 2003. *Philosophical Foundations of Neuroscience*. Malden, MA & Oxford: Blackwell.

Brockmeier, Jens. 1996. "Explaining the Interpretive Mind." *Human Development* 39: 287–295.

———. 2000. "Autobiographical Time." *Narrative Inquiry* 10 (1 Special Issue on Narrative Identity): 51–73.

———. 2009. "Stories to Remember: Narrative and the Time of Memory." *Storyworlds: A Journal of Narrative Studies* 1: 117–132.

———. 2010. "After the Archive: Remapping Memory." *Culture and Psychology* 16: 5–35.

———. 2012. "Narrative Scenarios: Toward a Culturally Thick Notion of Narrative." In *Oxford Handbook of Culture and Psychology*, edited by Jaan Valsiner, 439–467. Oxford & New York: Oxford University Press.

Bruner, Jerome. 1987. "The Transactional Self." In *Making Sense: The Child's Construction of the World*, edited by Jerome S. Bruner and H. Haste, 81–96. London & New York: Methuen.

———. 1990. *Acts of Meaning*. Cambridge: Harvard University Press.

Budson, Andrew E. 2011. "Memory Disfunction in Dementia." In *Handbook of Alzheimer's Disease and Other Dementias*, edited by Andrew E. Budson and Neil W. Kowall, 315–335. Hoboken, NJ: Wiley-Blackwell.

Butler, Judith. 1990. *Gender Trouble*. London & New York: Routledge.

Caddell, Lisa, and Linda Clare. 2010. "The Impact of Dementia on Self and Identity: A Systematic Review." *Clinical Psychology Review* 30: 113–128.

Clark, Andy. 2011. *Supersizing the Mind: Embodiment, Action, and Cognitive Extension*. Oxford & New York: Oxford University Press.

Clegg, David. 2010. Comment. In Bryce, Colette (Ed.), *Tell Mrs Mill her Husband is Still Dead*. The Trebus Project. Accessed 21 January 2014 https://sites.google.com/site/trebusprojects/projects-2/tell-mrs-mill-her-husband-is-still-dead.

Danziger, Kurt. 2008. *Marking the Mind: A History of Memory*. Cambridge: Cambridge University Press.

Dubois, Bruno, Harold H. Feldman, Claudia Jacova, et al. 2007. "Research Criteria for the Diagnosis of Alzheimer's Disease: Revising the NINCDS-ADRDA Criteria." *Lancet Neurology* 6: 734–746.

Edelman, Gerald. 2006. *Second Nature: Brain Science and Human knowledge*. New Haven, CT: Yale University Press.

Foucault, Michel. 1970. *The Order of Things: An Archaeology of the Human Sciences*. London: Tavistock.

Freeman, Mark. 2008. "Beyond Narrative: Dementia's Tragic Promise." In *Health, Illness and Culture: Broken Narratives*, edited by Lars-Christer Hydén and Jens Brockmeier, 169–184. New York and London: Routledge.

———. 2010. "Afterword: 'Even Amidst': Rethinking Narrative Coherence." In *Beyond Narrative Coherence*, edited by Matti Hyvärinen, Lars-Christer Hydén, Marja Saarenheimo, and Maria Tamboukou, 167–186. Amsterdam and Philadelphia: John Benjamins.

Gazzaniga, Michael S. 2006. *The Ethical Brain: The Science of our Moral Dilemmas*. New York: HarperPerennial.

———, R. B. Ivry, and G. R. Mangum, eds. 2009. *Cognitive Neuroscience: The Biology of the Mind*. New York & London: Norton.

Georgakopoulou, Alexandra. 2007. *Small Stories, Interaction and Identities*. Amsterdam & Philadelphia: John Benjamins.
Gergen, Kenneth J. 2010. "The Acculturated Brain." *Theory and Psychology* 20 (6): 795–816.
Goldstein, Kurt. 1934/1995. *The Organism: A Holistic Approach to Biology Derived from Pathological Data in Man*. New York: Zone Books.
Hacking, Ian. 1995. *Rewriting the Soul: Multiple Personality and the Sciences of Memory*. Princeton, NJ: Princeton University Press.
———. 1996. "Memory Science, Memory Politics." In *Tense Past: Cultural Essays in Trauma and Memory*, edited by P. Antze and M. Lambek, 76–88. New York: Routledge.
———. 2002. *Historical Ontology*. Cambridge: Harvard University Press.
Harré, Rom, and Grant Gillett. 1994. *The Discursive Mind*. Thousand Oaks, CA: Sage.
Hassabis, Demis, D. Kumaran, S. D. Vann, and Elenor Maguire. 2007. "Patients with Hippocampal Amnesia Cannot Imagine New Experiences." *Proceedings of the National Academy of Sciences USA* 104: 1726–1731.
———, and Elenor Maguire. 2007. "Deconstructing Episodic Memory with Construction." *Trends in Cognitive Sciences* 11: 299–306.
Herman, David. 2011. "Re-minding Modernism." In *The Emergence of Mind: Representations of Consciousness in Narrative Discourse in English*, edited by David Herman, 243–272. Lincoln: University of Nebraska Press.
Hydén, Lars-Christer. 2013. "Towards an Embodied Theory of Narrative and Storytelling." In *The Travelling Metaphor of Narrative*, edited by Matti Hyvärinen, Mari Hatavara, and Lars-Christer Hydén. Amsterdam & Philadelphia: John Benjamins.
Ingold, Timothy. 2012. Timothy Ingold on the Social Brain. *PLOS Neuroanthropology: Understanding the Encultured Brain and Body. September 3, 2012*. Accessed September 15, 2012. http://blogs.plos.org/neuroanthropology/2012/09/03/timothy-ingold-on-the-social-brain.
Jacova, Claudia. 2009. "Episodic Memory Tests in the Early Diagnosis of Alzheimer's Disease: The Index Study Experience." *Alzheimer's & Dementia* 5 (Supplement 4): 99.
———, Andrew Kertesz, Mervin Blair, John D. Fisk, and Harold H. Feldman. 2007. "Neuropsychological Testing and Assessment for Dementia." *Alzheimers & Dementia* 3 (4): 299–317.
Kitwood, Tom. 1997. *Dementia Reconsidered: The Person Comes first*. Buckingham, UK: Open University Press.
Klein, S. B., J. Loftus, and J. F. Kihlstrom. 2002. "Memory and Temporal Experience: The Effects of Episodic Memory Loss on an Amnesic Patient's Ability to Remember the Past and Imagine the Future." *Social Cognition* 20: 353–379.
Kontos, Pia. 2004. "Ethnographic Reflections on Selfhood, Embodiment and Alzheimer's Disease." *Ageing & Society* 24: 829–849.
Lindemann Nelson, Hilde. 2001. *Damaged Identities, Narrative Repair*. Ithaca & London: Cornell University Press.
Locke, John. (1690) 2008. *An Essay Concerning Human Understanding*. Oxford & New York: Oxford University Press.
Luria, Alexander. 1973. *The Working Brain: An Introduction to Neuropsychology*. New York: Basic Books.
Matthews, Eric. 2006. "Dementia and the Identity of the Person." In *Dementia: Mind, Meaning, and the Person*, edited by Julian C. Hughes, Stephen J. Louw, and Steven R. Sabat, 163–177. New York: Oxford University Press.
Medved, Maria I., and Jens Brockmeier. 2008. "Continuity Amid Chaos: Neurotrauma, Loss of Memory, and Sense of Self." *Qualitative Health Research* 18 (4): 469–479.
———. 2010. "Weird Stories: Brain, Mind, and Self." In *Beyond Narrative Coherence*, edited by Matti Hyvärinen, Lars-Christer Hydén, M. Saarenheimo, and Maria Tamboukou, 17–32. Amsterdam & Philadelphia: John Benjamins.
Michaelian, Kourken. 2010. "Is Memory a Natural Kind?" *Memory Studies* 4 (2): 170–189.
Nelson, Katherine. 2007. "Developing Past and Future Selves for Time Travel Narratives." *Behavioral and Brain Sciences* 30: 327–328.

Noë, Alva. 2009. *Out of our Heads*. New York: Hill & Wang.
Randall, W. L. 2011. "Memory, Metaphor, and Meaning: Reading for Wisdom in the Stories of Our Lives." In *Storying Later Life: Issues, Investigations, and Interventions in Narrative Gerontology*, edited by G. Kenyon, E. Bohlmeijer, and W. L. Randall, 20–38. Oxford & New York: Oxford University Press.
Ricoeur, Paul. 1992. *Oneself as Another*. Chicago: University of Chicago Press.
Rose, S. 2006. *The 21st-Century Brain: Explaining, Mending and Manipulating the Mind*. London: Vintage.
Sabat, Steven R. 2001. *The Experience of Alzheimer's Disease: Life through a Tangled Veil*. Oxford: Blackwell.
———. 2013. "The Person with Dementia as Understood through Stern's Critical Personalism." In *Beyond Loss: Dementia, Identity, Personhood*, edited by Lars-Christer Hyden, Hilde Lindemann Nelson, and Jens Brockmeier. Oxford & New York: Oxford University Press.
Schacter, Daniel. 1996. *Searching for Memory: The Brain, the Mind, and the Past*. New York: Basic Books.
———. 2002. *The Seven Sins of Memory: How the Mind Forgets and Remembers*. Boston: Houghton Mifflin.
———, D. R. Addis, and R. L. Buckner. 2008. "Episodic Simulation of Future Events: Concepts, Data, and Applications." *The Year in Cognitive Neuroscience, Annals of the New York Academy of Sciences* 1124: 39–60.
Singer, Wolf. 2006. "The Evolution of Culture from a Neurobiological Perspective." In *Evolution and Culture*, edited by S. C. Levinson and P. Jaisson, 181–201. Cambridge: MIT Press.
———. 2008. "The Brain: A Social Organ." *Die Zeit* 15: 39.
Sontag, Susan. 1978. *Illness as Metaphor*. New York: Farrar, Straus, & Giroux.
Spreng, R. N., R. A. Mar, and A. S. Kim. 2009. "The Common Neural Basis of Autobiographical Memory, Prospection, Navigation, Theory of Mind and the Default Mode: A Quantitative Meta-analysis." *Journal of Cognitive Neuroscience* 21: 489–510.
Stern, William. 1921. "Richtlinien für die Methodik der psychologischen Praxis (Guidelines for the Method of Psychological Praxis)." *Beihefte zur Zeitschrift für Angewandte Psychologie* 29: 1–16.
Suddendorf, Thomas, Donna R. Addis, and Michael Corballis. 2011. "Mental Time Travel and the Shaping of the Human Mind." In *Predictions in the Brain: Using our Past to Generate a Future*, edited by Moshe Bar, 344–354. Oxford & New York: Oxford University Press.
———, and Michael Corballis. 2007. "The Evolution of Foresight: What is Mental Time Travel, and is it Unique to Humans?" *Behavioral and Brain Sciences* 30: 299–351.
Szpunar, Karl. 2010. "Episodic Future Thought: An Emerging Concept." *Perspectives on Psychological Science* 5: 142.
———, J. C. K. Chan, and Kathleen McDermott. 2009. "Contextual Processing in Episodic Future Thought." *Cerebral Cortex* 19: 1539–1548.
———, and Endel Tulving. 2011. "Varieties of Future Experience." In *Predictions in the Brain: Using our Past to Generate a Future*, edited by Moshe Bar, 3–12. New York: Oxford University Press.
———, J. M. Watson, and Kathleen McDermott. 2007. "Neural Substrates of Envisioning the Future." *Proceedings of the National Academy of Sciences USA* 104: 642–647.
The Trebus Project. 2012. Accessed September 23, 2012. http://www.trebusprojects.org.
Tulving, Endel. 2002. "Chronesthesia: Awareness of Subjective Time." In *Principles of Frontal Lobe Function*, edited by D. T. Stuss and R. C. Knight, 311–325. New York: Oxford University Press.
Usita, P. M., I. E. Hyman, and K. C. Herman. 1998. "Narrative Intentions: Listening to Life Stories in Alzheimer's Disease." *Journal of Aging Studies* 12: 185–198.

6

Everyday Dramas: Comparing Life with Dementia and Acquired Brain Injury

MARIA I. MEDVED

As I begin writing this chapter, the provisional title for the collection in which it appears is *Beyond Loss*. This evocative title got me thinking about the words typically used to denote loss, words such as decline, deficit, and impairment. As a clinical neuropsychologist, I am all too intimately familiar with these words, especially as my instruments are designed to be "sensitive" to deficiencies. It also left me thinking about how patients and their families often struggle to translate abstract neuropsychological concepts about past, present, and future loss (and sometimes even recovery) into their everyday lives. It is, however, not only sufferers and their relations who encounter this problem. I do as well. These difficulties occur irrespective of whether the loss is due to injury, disorder, or disease.

This is not to say that the putative diagnosis does not play a role in the rendering of neuropsychological loss to lived reality and conversely, lived reality into neuropsychological loss. Diagnoses are of course associated with distinct normative story lines about what people might reasonably expect over the time continuum. But regardless of what type of cause underlies people's cognitive challenges, affected individuals and their families find the meaning of cognitive scores to be confusing. In addition, they and their families seem to draw on similar resources and strategies in their attempts to bring some clarity to the situation.

Nevertheless, medical professionals, and researchers in particular, treat people as straightforwardly categorizable on the basis of their neurological and neuropsychological profiles. For me, there is much that challenges this neurological segregation, which all but ignores the sociocultural processes undergirding the experience of disease or injury. One of the richest places to find evidence supporting this challenge is in the everyday life of the family as all members attempt to understand what it means for them to live with dementia or acquired brain injury.

With a view on persons and their families, I offer a comparative analysis that highlights the commonalities around the narrative meaning-making processes between a family where a member includes a person with dementia and another family with a person with acquired brain injury. Others have suggested that dementia is a brain disease that has interactional consequences similar to that of other brain disorders (Mates, Mikesell, and Smith 2010; Perkins 2007), and in this chapter this assertion is looked at more closely. I focus on two families as they attempt to interpret a small event—an event that is easily recognizable to people dealing with neurological challenges, a sort of everyday "drama"—by presenting and analyzing two excerpts, one from each family, taken from longer interviews. Before that, however, I offer a short overview of differences between and similarities across dementia and acquired brain injury.

Dementia and Acquired Brain Injury

Although it might seem easy to come up with a list of differences and similarities in relation to dementia and brain injury, it quickly becomes complicated. Even something that initially seems as clear-cut as different etiologies dissolves on closer examination. Take, for example, vascular dementia. Although it is considered a form of dementia, it is the result of repeated minor strokes so in a sense it is also a brain injury. This section is not meant to provide a comprehensive or detailed review but to serve as a general primer. I start with some general differences.

DIFFERENCES

Although the border between dementia and acquired brain injury is fuzzy, some overarching observations can be made (Table 6.1). The main difference between dementia and brain injury is that, generally, the former is often the result of a progressive brain disease, whereas the latter is the result of a brain insult. Depending on the type of dementia (e.g., Pick's or Alzheimer's disease), different parts of the brain are affected at differential rates, diffusely impacting many cognitive, and eventually, physical abilities. Acquired brain injury is most commonly the result of a traumatic brain injury, typically due to vehicular accidents or falls, strokes, or brain tumors (which are not mentioned further). In traumatic brain injury, neurons throughout the brain are stretched due to the sudden impact thus resulting in a diffuse injury. In stroke, the injury is considered focal in that

Table 6.1. **General differences between individuals with dementia and acquired brain injury**

Dementia	Acquired brain injury
Disease etiology	Injury etiology
Gradual change	Abrupt change
Neurodegeneration	Neuroregeneration
Diffuse	Localized/diffuse
Gradual physical change	Sudden physical change
Long-term trajectory is (relatively) certain	Long-term trajectory is uncertain (first years)
Geriatric (except for early onset)	Throughout the lifespan (traumatic brain injury younger, stroke older)
Identity maintenance/reformulation	Identity recovery/reformulation

the insult is confined to a certain area of the brain, which depends on where the vessel bleed or clot is located.

A precise etiology is important as it shapes the dementia illness or injury progression. Dementias, such as Alzheimer's disease, proceed over an extended period of time, in a process of relatively slow neurodegeneration that gradually leads to changes in cognitive, linguistic, and physical capabilities. It is important to remember, however, that there are significant individual differences in the progression and expression of these changes. They vary according to the extent to which one's environment is enriching and supportive (Bryan et al. 2011) as well as according to one's personal characteristics (e.g., Seiffert, Clare, and Harvey 2005).

In contrast, traumatic or vascular accidents occur at one point in time. From one moment to the next, one's brain, its habits, and the way one experiences oneself is suddenly transformed. Cognitive changes may be accompanied with physical ones (e.g., hemiparesis or hemiplegia, that is, reduced functioning on one side of the body). Due to the nature of injuries, they have the possibility of partial or full neuroregeneration or functional recovery. In contrast to the relatively "normative" biological course of dementia, the long-term prognoses for acquired brain injury patients remain uncertain, particularly for individuals left with primarily mild-to-moderate neuropsychological challenges. Beyond the generic observation that most of the healing occurs in the first two years and is more likely if the person is healthy and younger than forty years old, there are no obvious clues that indicate the future trajectory.

Suffice to say, the attempts by persons and families to come to terms with dementia and brain injury are interwoven with, throughout, and around an overriding set of narratives—either of hope or despair, of potential recovery, or certain decline. In dementia the thread of despair is coarser, harsher, whereas in acquired brain injury there is mostly a thread of hope, even if perhaps flickering and elusive. This does not mean there is no hope in people struggling with dementia or no despair in people dealing with brain injury (e.g., Antelius 2007; Soundy et al. 2013). After all, hope and despair are always in relation to something or some event, whether large or small, close or distant.

Needless to say, one of the main reasons for despair in dementia is related to the painful loss of one's precious memories and sense of who one is in the world. I revisit this idea in the similarities section. In the face of fading memories of one's self, family, and life, many researchers and clinicians have advocated memory books and the like (at least in the early stages) (Wilson and Glisky 2009). For the purposes of this chapter, it is enough to say that many of these approaches focus on buttressing the person's sense of self and identity, albeit often in a very individualistic and isolated way. In acquired brain injury, the emphasis is different in that it is on helping the person reformulate their sense of self and identity in a way that reflects their new circumstances. This is easier said than done, and even decades after their injury individuals with acquired brain injury mention they never regained a solid sense of self (e.g., Nochi 1998).

To close, a few words on sociodemographics. Although there is early onset dementia, most dementias arise when people are older. Generally the same is the case with stroke, although there is more variability in terms of age, with individuals in their forties and fifties also at risk. In terms of traumatic brain injury, the average age is much younger. Age differences have consequences, as younger and middle-age individuals are at the beginning or peak of their personal and professional life, and their brain injury may make it difficult to maintain relationships and hold steady employment. It has been documented that 70% of homeless people in North American suffered a traumatic brain injury before living on the streets (Hwang et al. 2008).

SIMILARITIES

Finding out that one has suffered, is suffering, or will suffer neurological changes is a highly traumatic event that shakes people to their very core (Table 6.2). Both dementia and acquired brain injury are met with a flood of intensely disorienting and fluctuating emotions: shock, sadness, anger and fear, and downright existential panic (Aminzadeh et al. 2007; Medved and Brockmeier 2008). It is well-known that affect such as anxiety and depression disorganizes thinking, so this makes it even more difficult for individuals and families to understand and adjust to what has happened, is happening, or will happen. It is not only disorganizing emotions

Table 6.2. **General similarities across dementia and acquired brain injury**

Dementia	Acquired brain injury
Loss (fear, grief, despair)	Loss (fear, grief, despair)
Hope	Hope
Decreased narrative ability	Decreased narrative ability (almost always)
Memory troubles	Memory troubles (almost always)
Relational context important	Relational context important
Conarration/scaffolding/care	Conarration/scaffolding/care
Preservation of personhood	Preservation of personhood
Struggle for agency	Struggle for agency
Altered sense of identity and self	Altered sense of identity and self
Interpretation of "dramas"	Interpretation of "dramas"

that persons with cognitive challenges have to cope with. On top of this, when they need it most, their individual ability to narrate has been lessened.

Narrative is one of the premier venues for making sense of our experiences. It offers an experiential space to weave together personal and medical concerns, where individuals can bind them into their life stories to figure out what their injury or disease might mean for them and what can be done about it. Without the capability to narrate, it is difficult for an individual to avert the "dissolution of the world and a shattering of his own self" (Goldstein 1995, 232) when under neurological stress.

As hard as it can be to get a handle on one's emotions without the organizing function of narrative, delineating a sense of self-identity in the context of neurological change is also knotty. Although I already mentioned identity issues in the difference section, this is one of those points not so easily categorized. The reason is that there is significant overlap in identity processes for persons with dementia or acquired brain injury. As people with dementia battle to hold onto past identities, so too do people with acquired brain injury. Just as people with acquired brain injury struggle to adjust their sense of self, so too do individuals with dementia.

A trial particular to individuals, whether they have dementia or brain injury, is dealing with memory loss in relation to identity, especially in Western cultures. Memory holds a very special place, originating with the belief that individual memories are needed for people to establish their identity as persons, as formulated paradigmatically by John Locke (Brockmeier, this volume). People who have memories assessed to be "vague," "confabulatory," and "inconsistent" not only have their recollections and viewpoints dismissed, but also their right to self-presentation and moral self-positioning. The implicit assumption is that an individual who has difficulty remembering their past is unable to define a sense of self or be agentic on this basis, and therefore does not need to (or even cannot) be given the right to full personhood, including the right to decide what they may or may not do.

Of great importance therefore is the social space in which one's memories and stories can be told to and reflected by others. In such interactive environments, people typically interpret and reinterpret events—remembered or not, shared or not—in forms of joint "conarration" (Ochs and Capps 2001; Medved and Brockmeier 2010). As Hydén points out, focusing on the person with the disorder as a participant engaged in interaction "help[s] us conceptualize the consequences of neurological disorders less as an individual problem but rather something that is dealt with in everyday interaction *together* with other persons" (Hydén, this volume). Furthermore, such acts of conarration are especially pivotal after neurotrauma because they bridge the cognitive gaps caused by the dementia or brain damage as others become the vicarious voice (Hydén 2008) for those who, as Randall (2009) puts it, need "narrative care."

Stories that emerge in such discursive conarrations contribute to how the person with cognitive disorders is viewed, that is, what rights and responsibilities they have, or more simply, what they may or may not do. Identity, personhood, and agency, thus, are not exclusively located in one's mind but also grounded in forms of action and interaction. This is clearly evidenced in the stories of two women and their families provided later in this chapter.

These social and cultural interactions are also fundamental for the rehearsal of stories that help patients and families understand the disease or injury. The role of narrative and discourse has been increasingly recognized as crucial to all partners involved in the illness or injury process, even healthcare providers (Hydén and Brockmeier 2008). Mattingly (1998, 2008) investigated how health professionals give meaning to patients' behavior, achievements, and dysfunctions in rehabilitation, in what she calls "healing dramas." These dramatic stories are molded into disease or injury narratives via "therapeutic emplotment," whereby events or dramas are arranged along a therapeutic plotline. Outside of the hospital, rehabilitation center, or day center the primary responsibility of emplotting everyday dramas into narratives, and conversely narratives into dramas, is left to families and patients.

Family

At home, people with dementia or brain injury and their families (or anyone else they might be in regular contact with) must interpret what events or "dramas" might mean. For family members, this task is surely fraught with more complexity than for external health providers because they have to find ways of reconciling the person they have known for a long time with what that person has become under the impact of dementia or a brain injury. How individual family members negotiate and understand such situations has consequences for everybody involved (Medved 2011; Perry and Olshansky 1996; Smith and Kobayashi 2002).

As seen in the interview excerpts of family conversations in this chapter, both dementia and brain injury bring with them far-ranging changes in the meanings attributed to activities and interactions by all people involved. Is this what is meant by "moderate" memory problems? Is it a "symptom"? Does it suggest that certain abilities are declining? Or perhaps improving (which is of course always hoped for after brain injuries)? More broadly, how should this, if at all, be emplotted into the larger medical narrative of the progression of disease or injury?

Families are typically immersed in an array of talk, comments, and reflections as they jointly try to understand what certain situations or events might mean. However, the attributed meanings are rarely equally shared among members. In countless acts of conarration, storylines are negotiated, accepted, and rejected (Bamberg 2011; Ochs and Capps 2001) with the net result that certain storylines are thickened and others are thinned. Another way to think about these multiple storylines is in terms of negotiation between narratives and counternarratives (Bamberg and Andrews 2004; Bamberg 2011), whereby individuals maneuver between and among different narrative threads.

To date, most clinical insight into family dynamics comes from the literature on dyadic relations, typically involving the primary caregiver and a person with cognitive difficulties exploring how they manage together (e.g., Clare and Shakespear 2004; Roger and Medved 2010; Ward-Griffin et al. 2007). This research, although extremely important, often sidelines family members who likewise have a stake in how shared and unshared family events are understood. It also narrows our view of persons with cognitive deficits by viewing them only in relation to one other person. Both Purves (2011; Purves and Phinney 2012/13) and Brewer (2005), for example, stress how studying family interaction provides a unique source for exploring how persons with dementia position themselves in broader interactional contexts and how other family members adjust to the changing identity of their loved one.

Dramas in the Family

The genesis of this section is research that involved interviewing families coping with dementia or brain injury. In analyzing the interview transcripts, I was struck by two stories about going shopping at a mall that seemed exceptionally similar. What was surprising is that one story came from a family with a person who has a brain injury and the other from a family with a person who has dementia. Before I proceed, I would like to mention that at the time of the interviews in question, I had known these families for about a year and the interviews were conducted around the kitchen table in their homes.

In each interview there was an instance where Ms P, who has brain injury, and Ms D, who has Alzheimer's disease, decided to go shopping for new clothes. Both took public transit to the mall and did not return until about six hours later. Both women were unable to say what occupied their time for all these hours and neither one left a note to inform their families where they had went, nor did they telephone home during their excursion. Most understandably, their families were worried. For each family, I provide some basic background information before offering a short excerpt from each interview followed by some analytic reflections.

MS P

At the time of the interview, Ms P was a fifty-six–year old divorced mother of two teenaged boys (aged thirteen and sixteen years) who had worked as a bank teller. Twelve months prior she was admitted to hospital for an aneurysm of the right communicating artery. She was primarily impacted by what has been assessed as "moderate" attention and memory impairments along with headaches and occasional dizziness. Since her aneurysm she has been unable to return to work. Ms P's siblings, who live in the same neighborhood, assist her with many everyday living activities, such as making sure she has enough food in the house. This is an extract from a longer interview, one in a series conducted with Ms P, her two sons, and her brother.

> Oldest Son: She's like independent now. But I mean, after the mall I told her, "you shouldn't be doing that" but now, I mean, like, I actually want her to go out by herself. I mean, she can do it. She goes to the doctor by herself, she goes to the bank by herself, she goes to the mall herself. So she's saying that people have to take her but she goes by herself all the time.
>
> Ms P: Oh, I can do things for myself. It depends on what I have to do. But there WAS that incident (referring to her shopping trip).
>
> Youngest Son: Ok, well, I think she's, she is 95% better. Right? But she's not how she was before she got sick, but she is basically the same, nothing has really changed… She can cook all the time now. She can clean…

>   Brother: My take on this is that there is no point in me getting her upset and letting her have it because I want her to go out. I want her to take that trip to venture out because that's a learning experience.
>
>   Oldest Son: It's like before she had the aneurysm and it's like your mom is home. Just like your mom is home full time now. I like it this way better than before when she was working cause you know, I have my Mom home and I have food when I come home from school.
>
>   Ms P: I do things on my own, like I cook, I clean. But I can't do much. I think I have to just take one day at a time and things will hopefully get easier and easier.

As the family converses, it becomes clear that the members attribute different meanings to the mall drama and use it to support different stories about Ms P. Although the oldest son begins by saying that Ms P shouldn't have gone to the mall on her own, he suddenly shifts his point of view and the incident becomes an illustration of his mother's recovery, rather than a marker of his mother's poor judgment or memory problems. The younger son's comments demonstrate a similar pattern; he maintains his mother is "not how she was before she got sick," but then he quickly shifts to "she is basically the same," in fact "95% better." Both vigorously buttress the argument that their mother has recovered with what they consider to be further evidence, namely, that she is fully capable of cooking and cleaning on her own.

Ms P's brother offers another interpretation. He sets out to say that there is still some learning his sister needs to do, but his view is halted from being further developed by the oldest son. Throughout the interview as a whole, Ms P's brother seems to be hesitant over what to think, perhaps wanting to protect the sons or be persuaded by the sons' narrative. Ms P herself also seems unclear about the meaning of the mall incident. She claims that she can go out "depending on what it is," but then she needs to take "one day at a time."

It is easy to speculate about the motivations underlying the sons' desire to put forth their version of their mother's recovery narrative; but more importantly it seems to me that through this discourse Ms P's recovery is translated into a "low" level of functioning. This interpretation leaves Ms P with little room to further recover. No doubt, involved here also is a gendered narrative: as long as Ms P can cook, clean, and go to the mall, she is fine, with no mentioning of her possibly returning to work. Although Ms P seems to comply with her sons' storyline throughout most of the interview, there are moments when she (and to a lesser extent her brother) offers a counternarrative, one in which she retains space for further recovery ("things will hopefully get easier and easier").

MS D

Ms D is a seventy-two–year old mother and wife diagnosed with Alzheimer's dementia two years prior to the interview, and is currently assessed to have "mild to moderate cognitive impairments." She currently lives with her seventy-four–year old husband and has two adult children, a daughter and son, both in their forties who live nearby. She worked part-time as a retail clerk but stopped working 11 years ago. Throughout her life she has been relatively healthy, only having minor ailments. At present, she primarily suffers from memory problems and some word-finding difficulties. Although she takes care of the house, she increasingly relies on her husband to help her out. She does not have a history of what the mainstream literature calls wandering.

> Son: She went out shopping for some new clothes on her own. She didn't tell anybody. She took the bus and made it to the mall but then got disoriented. You were out for hours and didn't even phone us to let us know where you were.
>
> Ms D: You're right. I, I should have called. Didn't think at the time. I got the skirt.
>
> Daughter: Maybe when you want to go shopping the next time, we can make it a girls' outing together, like the old days. We'll have coffee and stuff.
>
> Ms D: Very nice. I did find home again. I, I just had to take my time with people.
>
> Son: That's great mom. You did good, but why were you in the mall for hours?
>
> Husband: I panicked at the time and was about to call the police. I feel responsible because I went out for groceries. She's always been independent and stubborn (all laugh) and I want her to keep doing what she wants, but I just don't know, I just don't know. She got a nice pair of pants and she still does a lot of stuff around the house.
>
> Ms D: Yeah.

Again, as in the previous excerpt, different family members draw on the same event to offer different narratives. The son begins by recounting the event as if it was a shared one, by noting his mother made it to the mall but became disoriented. This is a plausible explanation, but by no means authoritative. Still, he presents it as an accurate reflection of what transpired, which leaves it to the others to challenge his recounting if they disagree. Implicit in his version is his view that the incident is a marker of his mother's cognitive decline; although, at the same time he does not absolve her of responsibility, in fact, he even seems to try to elicit some guilt ("you didn't even phone").

Even in the face of her son's rather convincing story, Ms D contests his interpretation by pointing to the hard evidence that she bought a skirt (actually, a pair of pants) and thus successfully achieved her goal; in doing so, she simultaneously engages in a face-saving maneuver in response to her sons' characterization that she therefore could not have been too disoriented. That she went on her own to the mall for hours without telling anyone is thus framed as a minor oversight.

Everybody in the family, including Ms D, senses that a directive is in the process of being formed: that she should no longer go shopping alone. Ms D's daughter softens this possible intervention by framing it as an open invitation to a "girls' day out." Ms D seems to accept this offer, but appears fully aware of the nature of this invitation and reasserts by saying that she just needs to "take [her] time with people" when on her own.

At this point, Ms D's husband enters the conversation, emphasizing his responsibility for the events and the decision at stake: it was he who left his wife alone and then "panick[ed]." In referring to what he sees as her personality characteristics—being independent and stubborn—he obviously tries to dedramatize her behavior and the situation. In the end, he seems to align himself with his wife, as if swayed by his wife's version, reiterating her continued capability to shop and engage in activities around the house. One narrative function of this discourse is that it delays his emergent role of "caregiver" and keeps the wife he knows around a bit longer.

Commonalities

As illustrated by Roach, Keady, and Bee and by Sabat (this volume), taking into account the distinctive histories and stories of each individual and domestic unit is an inseparable part of holistically understanding the family. Although there are idiosyncratic elements present in both families' talk interactions, there nevertheless appears to be some common narrative discursive processes between the families that seem connected to the unique constellation of biological, psychological, and social features that a neurological disorder such as dementia or brain injury brings with it. Some of these processes have also been observed in people with other diseases (Charmaz 1983), but as observed in the two small drama excerpts, the cognitive challenges present in neurological complaints gives them a distinct characterization.

To begin with, all members of both families use one event—the mall drama—as a marker of neuropsychological functioning, whether it is viewed as a sign of recovery, a disease symptom, or an indicator of stability. In dementia and after brain injury, the pull to interpret things through a neuropsychological lens seems irresistible. In the family including a person with dementia, the husband argues that the mall event means very little in terms of his wife's cognition, whereas the adult children situate the event in terms of cognitive loss and emplot it within a narrative of decline. Ms D's assessment of moderate impairment does not provide much clarity and the burden falls on families to figure out if and how cognition reveals itself, a process partially sorted through family dialogue among a corpus of small unremarkable stories about day-to-day events.

How family members construct and then interpret such events in terms of cognitive functioning has ramifications for the identity of everybody involved, but especially, of course, for the person with cognitive changes. For example, in the cognitive decline narrative of Ms D's children, her identity as a person with Alzheimer's disease gradually encroaches on her other identities and personal characteristics. As her identity as a person with dementia becomes progressively dominant, her autonomy and independence decreases in inverse proportion to her family's duty to provide additional attention, support, and care.

In the other family, the mall incident is used by the two teenage sons as evidence of their mother's almost total recovery from her brain injury—which would set the recovery bar seemingly quite low. In a sense, it even denies her status as a sufferer or, at least, downplays it and deprives her of a particular rehabilitation identity. This reading assumes that there are no further skills necessary to recover, and it also implies that the duty of others to provide care is no longer required. At the same time, it gives her the autonomy and the right, at least theoretically, to carry out whatever activities she sees fit.

This is not to say that the teenage boys' mother, although in a narratively vulnerable position due to her neurological injury, just passively takes over their interpretation. As demonstrated in the excerpts, both women were actively involved in the family interactions, contesting certain stories and elaborating others. They did so in a manner that demonstrated ongoing awareness of how others view and "narrativize" them. Ms D, the woman with dementia, energetically opposed the emergence of a reductive narrative; she was also keen to preserve her social standing and engaged in face-saving maneuvers to do so. Ms P, the woman with the brain injury, brings the mall drama into discursive play to make the case that she still has some recovering to do.

What I found striking in these family conversations was how both women provided pragmatic, sensible reflections on their own cognitive functioning, good examples of counternarratives. Ms D observes she can still do things albeit with support from others. Ms P observes that she needs to take it "one day at a time." It is not a stretch to view these expressions as drawing on bits of medical discourse that might have been taken over from health professionals. The point here is that these expressions are aptly, almost expertly, inserted into the ongoing conversation. Even more surprising, Ms P, although neuropsychological assessments frame her as someone with "memory problems," is left to point out her "limitations," remembering what others seem to have forgotten, or want to forget.

The final commonality I would like to point out is that both families are grappling with issues related to time. Due to the different medical trajectories associated with dementia and brain injury, the two families have a very different relationship with it, but nevertheless, family talk is very much about the past, present, and future. At this point, it bears keeping in mind that the families are in the midst of interpreting their experiences and their accounts are far from complete or stable. I am not implying that families be encouraged to settle on just one narrative, not only because it simply is too difficult to know what narrative is the best fit. There also is another reason: leaving space for multiple narratives within the family often serves an important function because it "subjunctivizes" illness or injury narratives. Good and Good (1994) have observed this for individual storytelling, and I have shown how multiple narratives can serve to open possibilities for "empowerment, social support, and hope" for an entire family.

This is particularly obvious with respect to how both families use time as a discursive resource for the creation of hope (or lack thereof). In one family, the sons' story is meant to optimistically restore the past, where a return to pre–brain injury functioning is possible and in effect, has almost already been accomplished. This, in essence, deletes the brain injury; it thus bears resemblance to Frank's (1995) restitution narrative. Diverging from this temporal trajectory, Ms P feels uneasy with the foreclosed temporality of her sons' narrative, as she wants to inhabit the future, a future where, hopefully, further recovery is possible and indeterminant.

Although "restitution" to the past may be desperately desired by all members of Ms D's family, it is not an interpretative option. Instead, the emerging family narrative, at least of Ms D's adult children, is a story that prepares for the future and situates the protagonists in a future where their mother no longer can function. Here time has lost its openness and possibilities, along with hope. Although this future focus may be eminently practical, it forecloses her future and also erases the present of Ms D. She thus objects to this putative erasure particularly since it undervalues her present achievement, that she *can* currently shop, and her narrative of immediacy (which is linked with the establishment of hope in the present) is negated.

Notwithstanding, what is curious is that Ms D wants to stay in the present, yet the basis of many clinical interventions to increase life satisfaction, such as family reminiscence therapy (e.g., Savundranayagam, Dilley, and Basting 2011), are geared to exactly that, helping the person with dementia remain in the present.

Perhaps in certain cases, although often framed as helping the person with the diagnosis, such interventions are needed more for family members and others than for persons like Ms D. Yet, it seems that the aim should be to help everyone stay in the present *together*.

Final Remarks

This chapter emerged out of my difficulties explaining what neuropsychological test scores might mean to persons with neurological disorders and their families in the context of their everyday life. Some of these difficulties have to do with the assumptions behind neuropsychological testing and assessment practices, such as viewing cognitive capacities as decontextualized from the environment (this not only includes "symptoms" but also the capacity to figure out what these "symptoms" are) and neglecting the significance of the agency of the persons with dementia or brain injury. But what struck me, translation difficulties aside, is how similar patients and families are in their attempts to understand cognitive changes, drawing on similar narrative-discursive resources and strategies and negotiating narratives and counternarratives in spite of different neurological issues.

To close this chapter I would like to elaborate on the practice of categorizing people on the basis of their neurological profiles. Reviewing the general differences between persons with dementia and acquired brain injury (Table 6.1), it becomes obvious that many of the listed points are related to biological factors, factors on which afflicted individuals and their families typically have minimal influence. In contrast, if the table for similarities across people with dementia or acquired brain injury is consulted (Table 6.2), we see that most of the points relate to psychological and social factors, factors on which the persons with the disorder and their families have relative control and which they can actively influence. This is amply demonstrated by the interactions in the families, which ultimately could be listed in the table in terms of narrative-discursive strategies. These strategies may be subtle, but their influence on agency, identity, and personhood is large. It is here where people *can* move beyond loss.

In conducting research based on difference that is defined by neurological disorders, we explicitly give precedence to biology, even if our intent may be to articulate an alternative, less deterministic perspective. In conducting research based on similarity, the end result is to prioritize the psychological and social context in which persons with disorders live. Comparative analysis can help break down the all too common "silo approach" and help us hone in on what is unique or shared and what is more or less changeable or immutable. This approach promises to be a fruitful adjunct to better understand people with dementia *and* acquired brain injury, as well as individuals with other neurological issues, such as intellectual disabilities. I am not arguing that biological etiologies and neuropsychological trajectories do not have a major impact on the issues at stake (they most obviously do), but rather that comparative analysis adds something essential, helping us reframe our work in a nuanced and holistic way by being aware of the crucial importance of the social and cultural life of persons and families rather than simply their brains.

References

Aminzadeh, Faranak, Anna Byszewksi, Frank Molnar, and Marg Eisner. 2007. "Emotional Impact of Dementia Diagnosis: Exploring Persons with Dementia and Caregivers' Perspectives." *Aging and Mental Health* 11 (3): 281–290.

Antelius, Elenor. 2007. "The Meaning of the Present: Hope and Foreclosure in Narrations About People with Severe Brain Damage." *Medical Anthropology Quarterly* 21 (3): 324–342.

Bamberg, Michael. 2011. "Narrative Practice and Identity Navigation." In *Varieties of Narrative Analysis*, edited by James A. Holstein and Jaber F. Gubrium. London: Sage Publications.

Bamberg, Michael, and Molly Andrews, eds. 2004. *Considering Counter-Narratives: Narrating, Resisting, Making Sense*. Philadelphia: John Benjamins Publishing Company.

Brewer, Jeutonne. 2005. "Carousel Conversation: Aspects of Family Roles and Topic Shift in Alzheimer's Talk." In *Alzheimer Talk, Text, and Context*, edited by Boyd H. Davis. Basingstoke, UK: Palgrave Macmillan.

Bryan, James, Patricia Boyle, Aron Buchman, Lisa Barnes, and David Bennett. 2011. "Life Space and the Risk of Alzheimer Disease, Mild Cognitive Impairment, and Cognitive Decline in Old Age." *Geriatric Psychiatry* 19 (11): 961–969.

Charmaz, Kathy. 1983. "Loss of Self: A Fundamental Form of Suffering in the Chronically Ill." *Sociology of Health and Illness* 5 (2): 168–195.

Clare, Linda, and Pam Shakespeare. 2004. "Negotiating the Impact of Forgetting." *Dementia* 3 (2): 211–232.

Frank, Arthur. 1995. *The Wounded Storyteller: Body, Illness and Ethics*. Chicago: University of Chicago Press.

Goldstein, Kurt. [1934] 1995. *The Organism: A Holistic Approach to Biology Derived from Pathological Data in Man*. New York: Zone Book.

Good, Byron, and Mary-Jo Vecchio Good. 1994. "The Subjunctive Mode: Epilepsy Narratives in Turkey." *Social Science and Medicine* 38 (6): 835–842.

Hwang, Stephen, Angela Colantonio, Shirley Chiu, George Tolomiczenko, Alex Kiss, Laura Cowan, Donald Redelmeier, and Wendy Levinson. 2008. "The Effect of Traumatic Brain Injury on the Health of Homeless People." *Canadian Medical Association Journal* 179 (8): 779–784.

Hydén, Lars-Christer. 2008. "Vicarious Voices." In *Culture, Health and Illness: Broken Narratives*, edited by Lars-Christer Hydén and Jens Brockmeier. New York: Routledge Press.

Hydén, Lars-Christer and Jens Brockmeier. 2008. "From the Retold to the Performed story: Introduction." In *Health, Illness and Culture: Broken Narratives*, edited by. Lars-Christer Hydén and Jens Brockmeier. New York: Routledge.

Mates, Andrea, Lisa Mikesell, and Michael Sean Smith, editors. 2010. *Language, Interaction, and Frontotemporal Dementia: Reverse Engineering the Social Mind*. London: Equinox.

Mattingly, Cheryl. 1998. *Healing Dramas and Clinical Plots: The Narrative Structure of Experience*. New York: Cambridge University Press.

Medved, Maria I. 2011. "Recovered or Recovering: Negotiating Rehabilitation After Stroke." *Topics in Stroke Rehabilitation* 18 (1): 35–39.

Medved, Maria I., and Jens Brockmeier. 2008. "Talking About the Unthinkable: Brain Injuries and the Catastrophic Reaction." In *Culture, Health and Illness: Broken Narratives*, edited by Lars-Christer Hydén and Jens Brockmeier. New York: Routledge.

Medved, Maria I., and Jens Brockmeier. 2008. "Continuity Amidst Chaos: Neurotrauma, Loss of Memory and Sense of Self." *Qualitative Health Research* 18: 469–479.

Medved, Maria I., and Jens Brockmeier. 2010. "Weird Stories: Brain, Mind, and Self." In *Beyond Narrative Coherence*, edited by Matti Hyvarinen, Lars-Christer Hyden, and Maria Tamboukou. Philadelphia: John Benjamins.

Nochi, Masahiro. 1998. "'Loss of Self' in the Narratives of People with Traumatic Brain Injuries: A Qualitative Analysis." *Social Science and Medicine* 46: 869–878.

Ochs, Elinor, and Lisa Capps. 2001. *Living Narrative: Creating Lives in Everyday Storytelling*. Cambridge, MA: Harvard University Press.

Perkins, Michael. 2007. *Pragmatic Impairment*. Cambridge: Cambridge University Press.

Perry, JoAnn and Ellen Olshanky. 1996. "A Family's Coming to terms with Alzheimer's Disease." *Western Journal of Nursing of Research*. 18(1): 12–28.

Purves, Barbara. 2011. "Exploring Positioning in Alzheimer Disease Through Analyses of Family Talk." *Dementia* 10: 35–58.

Purves, Barbara, and Alison Phinney. 2012/13. "Family Voices: A Family Systems Approach to Understanding Communication in Dementia." *Canadian Journal of Speech-Language Pathology and Audiology* 36 (4): 284–298.

Randall, William. 2009. "The Anthropology of Dementia: A Narrative Perspective." *International Journal of Geriatric Psychiatry* 24: 322–324.

Roger, Kerstin, and Maria I. Medved. 2010. "Couples Manage Change in the Case of Terminal Medical Conditions Including Neurological Decline." *International Journal of Qualitative Studies on Health and Well-Being* 5 (2): 5129. doi: 10.3402/qhw.v5i2.5129.

Savundranayagam, Marie Y., Lorna J. Dilley, and Anne Basting. 2011. "StoryCorps' Memory Loss Initiative: Enhancing Personhood for Storytellers with Memory Loss." *Dementia* 10 (3): 415–433.

Seiffert, Anna, Linda Clare, and Richard Harvey. 2005. "The Role of Personality and Coping Style in Relation to Awareness of Currently Functioning in Early-Stage Dementia." *Aging and Mental Health* 9 (6): 535–541.

Smith, André and Karen Kobayashi. 2002. "Making Sense of Alzheimer's Disease in an Intergenerational Context: The Case of a Japanese Canadian Nsei (Second-Generation) Headed Family." *Dementia* 1(2): 213–225.

Soundy, Andrew, Brent Smith, Helen Dawes, Hardev Pall, Katrina Gimbrere, and Jill Ramsay. 2013. "Patient's Expression of Hope and Illness Narratives in Three Neurological Conditions: A Meta-Ethnography." *Health Psychology Review* 7(2): 177–201. doi: 10.1080/17437199.2011.568856.

Ward-Griffin, Catherine, Abram Oudshoorn, Kristie Clark, and Nancy Bol. 2007. "Mother–Adult Daughter Relationships within Dementia Care: A Critical Analysis." *Journal of Family Nursing* 13 (1): 13–32.

Wilson, Barbara, and Elizabeth Glisky. 2009. *Memory Rehabilitation: Integrating Theory and Practice*. New York: Guildford Press.

7

Musical Embodiment, Selfhood, and Dementia

PIA C. KONTOS

Henry Dryer lives in a nursing home and mostly sits slumped over the tray attached to his wheelchair with his arms folded. He has dementia. He doesn't speak, and rarely moves. Then a personal support worker puts headphones on him attached to an iPod with his favorite music, and with the music Henry begins to shuffle his feet, his folded arms rock back and forth, his face assumes expression, his eyes open wide, and he is totally animated by the music. His animation does not cease when the headphones are removed. Henry, normally silent and virtually unable to answer the simplest "yes" and "no" questions, is quite voluble; when asked what his favorite music was when he was young, he responds "Cab Calloway" and breaks into Calloway-style scat talking. This is followed by a soulful rendition of what he says is his favorite Calloway song—"I'll be Home for Christmas."

Henry's performance features in an extraordinarily moving rough cut of a documentary. *Alive Inside* (Rossato-Bennett 2012), produced by Michael Rossato-Bennett, follows social worker Dan Cohen who creates personalized iPod playlists for people in elder care facilities with various conditions, especially those, like Henry, with dementia. The project is devoted to improving quality of life by reconnecting residents of long-term care with the music they love. The director posted the clip of Henry on YouTube prior to the premiere of the film, and in just four days it was viewed by three million people. The YouTube clip received vast media coverage, including attention from *USA Today*; the *Wall Street Journal*; the *Washington Post*; ABC News; the *LA Times*; the *Guardian*; and news organizations in Brazil, Canada, and Pakistan.

Henry's musicality has captivated the world. Yet reports of the evidence of musicality in dementia (Cuddy and Duffin 2005; Pickles and Jones 2006), as in the case of Henry, suggest that despite even advanced stages of dementia, it is not a rare phenomenon to retain musical ability. Malcolm Pointon, a talented pianist, composer, and music lecturer from Thriplow, England, offers another compelling case of musical intelligence despite his diagnosis of probable Alzheimer's disease at the early age of fifty-one.

After the diagnosis, Malcolm's wife Barbara decided to allow film-maker Paul Watson to document their journey with Alzheimer's disease on film (Watson 1999), which took place over the course of eleven years. When Malcolm first started to experience memory problems he recorded his early symptoms in his diary—"thoughts and actions slipping from my grasp"; "fog like experience clouds the words I am writing"; "aching back, feet and legs"; "very strong vivid attack of the vision, don't tell anyone"; "very forgetful, lacking in confidence"; "tendency to panic." Barbara recounts in the film how the progressing illness interfered with Malcolm's daily tasks—he often would confuse the proper setting of table cutlery; he drove to Cambridge where he frequently would go to change his tires and got lost, returning in a panic; his speech was often incoherent; and he progressively needed more and more assistance with washing and dressing.

Yet when Malcolm was severely demented in terms of standardized psychometric tests, scoring zero on most, he was still able to improvise music fluently. Long after he lost the ability to read music and write down his own compositions in conventional notation he continued to improvise on the piano and even spontaneously with makeshift instruments. There is a scene in the film where Malcolm is sharing lunch with his son, himself a drum musician who plays jazz and rock. Conversation is a challenge for Malcolm, who stumbles with word-finding issues and has difficulties staying focused. Spontaneously he begins to tap his plate with his fingers as if playing a keyboard. His son joins him by tapping his own plate, using his index fingers as drum sticks. Malcolm continues to improvise free jazz by introducing new sounds and more complex rhythms, coordinating the tapping of his knife on his glass and then his plate. Then, as if the knife were a keyboard, he plays it with his right hand allowing it to tap against his plate, keeping a clear regular meter. Malcolm focuses intensely on his playing, tilting his head and bringing his ear close to the table as if to more acutely discern sound and rhythm. The two continue to improvise in this way for several intense minutes, all the while keeping a strongly pulsed rhythm.

Even after Malcolm stopped playing—either because he no longer felt able to or because of increasing stiffness in his wrists—his wife Barbara noted that listening to music still wholly engaged his attention (Pickles and Jones 2006). With verbal communication gone, she observed that music still played a very large part in his daily life. Despite that he became immobile, mute, unable to process what he saw, doubly incontinent, and had difficulties with autonomic systems, such as swallowing, Barbara described his response to music: "He no longer recognizes me as his wife... but, amazingly, he recognizes pieces of music which mean a lot to him and a tear will trickle down his face. When a familiar piece of music is played, his eyes no longer look vacantly into space—they widen and take on a brightness and appearance of concentration—even looking towards the source of the sound" (Pickles and Jones 2006, 89).

According to conventional explanations of music perception, the measure of music's importance is its cognitive efficacy (Bowman 2004). Yet how can recourse to mental processes account for Henry's and Malcolm's musicality given their dementia? Their continued musicality is further perplexing given that Alzheimer's disease and its kindred dementias are usually described and analyzed in terms of an assumed existential outcome: the loss of self with the concomitant erosion of individual agency (Herskovitz 1995; Ronch 1996).

It is the central aim of this chapter to explore how an alternative perspective on music perception—one of embodied selfhood—brings a new and critical dimension to the discourse on music, and, more broadly, the implicit assumption that selfhood depends exclusively upon cognition. I have chosen the cases of Henry and Malcolm because they raise crucial questions about agency, intentionality, and selfhood, which form the focus of my analysis.

Conventional Approaches to Music Perception

The dominant paradigm of music perception is linguistic and propositional in nature. Theories to explain musical intelligence are largely premised upon information-processing models that reduce music perception to a sophisticated stimulus-response system, rendered musical by mental manipulation of lower-order stimuli (Bowman 2004). The implicit assumption is that music perception is cognitive. Without such cognitive intervention—transformation, processing, representation of lower-order stimuli and auditory sense data—the assumption, argues Bowman, is that music would be perceived as little more than "a booming, buzzing confusion" (2004, 9). But can we understand Henry's and Malcolm's musical engagement in terms of an abstract mental pattern construction, accomplished by the same cognitive mechanism as linguistic, propositional discourse?

Understandings about musical intelligence implicit in conventional accounts derive from a presumed dichotomy between mind and body, and an inherent inferiority of bodily constituted knowledge (Bowman 2004). Theorists have sought to locate music's value in its abstract, mindful, and cognitively distinguished benefits, from which bodily perception and production are jettisoned as distraction or contaminants (Bowman 1998). Where music's distinctive origin in bodily experience is explicitly acknowledged, such experience is reduced to low-level auditory processing and is of interest only to the extent that it feeds into and enables higher-level, language-like, rational/inferential processes. The body and its materiality, subjectivity, temporality, and specificity are subjugated to characteristics deemed durable, objective, structural, and ideal (Bowman 2004). Consequently corporeality, as a potential source of agency, has largely been neglected in the discourse on musical intelligence and explorations of the subjective experience of music (Bowman and Powell 2007). Even the field of music and emotion is largely dominated by evolutionary and neuropsychological frameworks with a focus on the cognitive organization of musical experience (Juslin and Sloboda 2001).

The habit of treating the body as the subordinated counterpart of mind is difficult to change. While there have been important strides made in delivering music from the vagaries of cognitive science (Bowman 2004; Bowman and Powell 2007; Elliott 1991; Maus 2010; Shusterman 2010), bodily constituted knowledge is still cast in terms of "the minded body" (see for example Bowman 2004), or in terms of brain-body-world interactions, without sufficiently elaborating the foundational aspects of nonrepresentational intentionality (Gibbs 2005).

Thus, despite noble efforts to rethink intelligence and cognition, reference to the mind effectively reproduces the dichotomous structure that analyses are intended to transcend. A further limitation is that even where bodily roots of musical experience are theorized more fully in terms of their nonrepresentational nature (see for example Holgersen 2010), the interrelationship between prereflective intentionality and selfhood is left woefully unaddressed. In the context of the disparate and discursive literature on Alzheimer's disease and other dementias that assume the erasure of selfhood with advancing cognitive impairment, such inattention is particularly egregious.

The Naturalization of Musical Cognition

The subjugation of the body in music perception can be traced to classical aesthetic theory where music's value is said to arise from aesthetic experience rooted in refined perceptual sensibilities (see Bowman's discussion of Alperson, Hegel, and Deweyan in Bowman and Powell 2007, 2–3). The mind-centered and mind-contained approach to music perception has also been traced to the cognitivist paradigm that has long dominated cognitive science and that defines the context within which the field of music has sought to explain its significance (Bowman 2004). Yet attention to the deep-seated philosophical roots of the submergence of the body problematizes in important ways the naturalization of cerebral accounts of music perception. Of significance here is the seventeenth-century rise of the "modern self" where the self and brain became consubstantial (Vidal 2009), with the implicit subordinate role assigned to corporeality. As Vidal has argued, this ideology of the self—"the individualism characteristic of western and westernized societies, the supreme value given to the individual as autonomous agent of choice and initiative, and the corresponding emphasis on interiority" (2009, 7)—treats the brain as the organ responsible for the functions with which the self is identified. The constructed nature of the "cerebral subject" (Ortega 2009; Vidal 2009) is even further apparent given historical discontinuities in how the self is conceptualized. The modern treatment of the self is in striking contrast to the Aristotelian notion of materiality and signification (Aristotle 1991), which implies an essential corporeality of the self (Kontos 2004b).

The cerebral subject has acquired a presumed "ontological preeminence" (Vidal 2009, 426) that is founded upon the socially constructed brain-self consubstantiality. The naturalization of brain-self coupling is critical, since it is implicated in the formation and practice of dehumanizing persons with dementia (Kontos 2004a, 2005, 2006); the self is thought to be increasingly devoid of content with cognitive impairment, a process that has been referred to as "unbecoming" a self (Fontana and Smith 1989), and a "drifting towards the threshold of unbeing" (Kitwood and Bredin 1992, 285). Cohen and Eisdorfer (1986, 22), commenting on their many years of working with people with Alzheimer's disease and their families, maintain that "the victim of Alzheimer's must eventually come to terms with...the complete loss of self." Davis (2004, 375) echoes these sentiments by maintaining that "what is so devastating about the relentless nature of dementia is the very splintering of the sedimented layers of Being," until ultimately "there is nothing left."

But if the very notion of dementia implies the destruction of selfhood, how do we explain musical intelligence, as captured in the cases of Henry and Malcolm? Might musical performance in the face of the progression of Alzheimer's disease reside somewhere deeper than cognition? I wish to explore a noncerebral notion of selfhood—"embodied selfhood" (Kontos 2004a, 2005, 2006)—in the context of music perception in dementia. Embodied selfhood, which here I extend to the "musical self" (Pickles and Jones 2006, 74), is premised on a prereflective notion of agency that resides below the threshold of cognition, and facilitates meaningful engagement with the world. I shall argue that the key to the seemingly inexplicable coherent and spontaneous expressions of musicality that emerge from the depths of dementia is to be found in the body's own primordial potential and sociocultural significance that sustain selfhood at a prereflective level (Kontos 2004a, 2005, 2006).

Embodied Selfhood

Embodied selfhood is premised on a prereflective notion of agency that resides below the threshold of cognition and is manifest primarily in corporeal ways.[1] As an embodied dimension of human existence, selfhood persists even with severe dementia, as demonstrated, for example, in religious and artistic practices (Kontos 2006), aversion to particular foods (Kontos, Miller, and Mitchell 2010; Kontos et al. 2010), and bodily dispositions that convey the prior vocation (Kontos and Naglie 2007a; Kontos, Miller, and Mitchell 2010; Kontos and Naglie 2007b) of persons with dementia. This is not to suggest that embodied selfhood encapsulates all aspects of selfhood. Indeed these embodied self-expressions do not constitute the whole of what persons with dementia once were (Matthews 2006). Yet, shifting the discourse on selfhood in Alzheimer's disease toward a greater recognition of the way humans are embodied offers a new lens through which to explore the coherent and spontaneous expressions of musicality that are observed to emerge from the depths of dementia.

Embodied selfhood takes its theoretical bearings from Merleau-Ponty's understanding of nonrepresentational or basic intentionality (Merleau-Ponty 1962) and from Bourdieu's concept of habitus, which links bodily dispositions to structures of the social world (Bourdieu 1977, 1990). It is by extending Merleau-Ponty's and Bourdieu's theoretical perspectives on the body that I advance an embodied perspective on selfhood, with selfhood understood in terms of the primordial and sociocultural sources of the agency of the body.

More specifically, I conceptualize Merleau-Ponty's elucidation of basic intentionality as providing the corporeal foundation of selfhood evidenced by the existential expressiveness of the body. Merleau-Ponty's basic intentionality is the body's concrete, spatial, and prereflective directedness toward the lived world. It refers to a field of possible movements, a kind of inner map of movements, that the body naturally "knows" how to perform without having to reflect upon such movements. In Merleau-Ponty's words, "a system of possible movements... radiates from us to our environment" (1964, 5), giving us at every moment a practical and implicit hold on our body, a hold that situates us as subjects perceptually, linguistically, as well as through motor activity. In this "system of possible movements," the body possesses, according to Merleau-Ponty, a coordinating capacity in relation to itself through what he refers to as the "primary perceptual" level that is prior to explicit intellection. I understand the primacy of perception as providing the foundation for selfhood and therefore argue that selfhood, at the most fundamental level, must be understood as inhering in the existential capacity of the body to engage with the world (Kontos 2004a, 2006).

In Merleau-Ponty's discussion of basic intentionality, he makes no reference to sociocultural modes of expression because his exclusive concern is with capacity per se. However, clearly there is a sociocultural style or content to bodily movements and gestures, the source of which cannot be attributed to a primary level of signification. Bourdieu's concept of habitus is pertinent here because it foregrounds the sociocultural sources of bodily practices.

Bourdieu's sociological approach to understanding the embodiment of social structures further informs my articulation of embodied selfhood in that I conceptualize habitus as instilling at a prereflective level the sociocultural dispositions of selfhood. Our social being derives from habitus, which Bourdieu defines as socialized inclinations that are associated with membership in a particular cultural group and that instill in individuals dispositions and generative schemes for being and perceiving (Bourdieu 1977, 1990). Habitus comprises dispositions and forms of know-how that are learned by the body but cannot be explicitly articulated. It is a form of knowledge that does not pass through consciousness, for it is enacted at a prereflective level. As Bourdieu states, "the schemes of the *habitus*...owe their specific efficacy to the fact that they function below the level of consciousness and language, beyond the reach of introspective scrutiny or control by the will" (1984, 466). Just as dispositions are embodied and materialized in practice, so is selfhood embodied and manifested in socioculturally specific ways of being-in-the-world (Kontos 2004a).

The Primordial Depths of Music

For Merleau-Ponty, perception is a *prereflective* intercourse with the world. Existential understanding is prior to and independent of reflective thought. It is not a proposition of the form "I think that," but rather a practical form of "I know how," which is in no way dependent upon language. Practical consciousness represents that inarticulate but fundamental attunement to things, which is our being-in-the-world (1962, 79). That attunement is a function of bodily schema, the body's natural investment with a certain perceptual significance, a bodily know-how or practical sense. Thus, in reference to Merleau-Ponty's notion of nonrepresentational intentionality, music perception is understood not in cognitive terms but rather as coming into being by taking for granted "all the latent knowledge of itself that...[our] body possesses" (1962, 233). This latent knowledge can be understood as "kinesthetic background" (116), with musical gesture and its background both being "moments of a unique totality" (110). The background to the gesture, or its form, is not related by way of being a representation that is externally linked, but rather is immanent in the gesture itself, impelling and sustaining it at every moment.

The fact that musical performance is a learned activity in no way lessens the significance of the primordial potentiality of the body that is engaged. Merleau-Ponty himself uses the example of typing, another activity that is learned, in order to emphasize the prereflective nature of the body. In other words, Merleau-Ponty wishes to argue that the primordial body is operative in the same way whether or not the activity is learned. Merleau-Ponty describes one who knows how to type without having to think out the location of each letter on the keyboard (1962, 144). Even more than this, although the typist does not know where the keys are in a reflective sense, the typist, to make any attempt to provide a reflective and discursive account of the keyboard layout, would have to imagine typing in order to see the direction in which his or her fingers move to hit the appropriate keys. Knowledge of typing, Merleau-Ponty argues, is in the hands and manifests itself only when bodily effort is made and cannot be articulated in detachment from that effort. Merleau-Ponty here does not intend for knowledge to be understood in an intellectualist fashion where it would be associated with the supposedly self-transparent activities of a reflexive subject. Indeed, the kind of knowledge the typist has of the keyboard is a practical, embodied knowledge, quite remote and distinct from discursive knowledge. Knowledge, as Merleau-Ponty understands it here, is the capacity for acting, the know-how belonging to a subject whose primary relation to the environment is that of prereflective, active, and practical involvement.

These elucidations displace the primacy of cognitive consciousness and underscore the significance of bodily, or embodied, consciousness (Kontos 2003). In so doing they enable us to more clearly understand that Henry's and Malcolm's ability to engage in musicality is completely dependent upon having incorporated the music into their bodily schema, just as the typist incorporates the keyboard space into their bodily schema. The resilience of musical expression can thus be understood in terms of embodied know-how and practical sense, that is, a perspectival grasp of the world from "the point of view" of the body. Their musical expression is founded upon bodily intentionality that is distinct from the self-transparent activities of a reflexive subject. Musical engagement then is not the function of a cognitive form of consciousness that carries the body to a given space by way of a strategic plan formulated beforehand. It is a bodily form of consciousness, what in Merleau-Ponty's terms is the body's prereflective ability to direct itself toward the world.

The persistence of musicality despite advanced Alzheimer's disease exemplifies the existential expressiveness of the body that I argue is a fundamental source of selfhood (Kontos 2004a, 2005, 2006). Selfhood as an expression of musicality should be understood as the unique synthesis of movement and embodied perception that, according to Merleau-Ponty, is dependent upon the body's ability to seize and transform the perceptible into something meaningful (Merleau-Ponty 1962). Yet, the primordial basis for musical expression is but half the picture. Bowman has argued about musical experience that "skillful actions and performances are always also cultural" (2004, 23). There is a sociocultural origin to musical preferences that is not attributable to a primary level of signification and that shapes bodily proclivities and dispositions. Bourdieu's concept of *habitus* is pertinent here because it foregrounds the sociocultural sources of bodily practices that can inform our understanding of the ways in which embodiment and enculturation are coimplicated.

The Sociocultural Logic of the Musical Body

Bourdieu's sociological approach to understanding the embodiment of social structures further informs my analysis of the musical self in dementia in that I conceptualize habitus as instilling at a prereflective level the sociocultural dispositions of selfhood. Our social being derives from habitus, what Bourdieu defines as socialized inclinations, associated with membership in a particular cultural group, which instill in individuals dispositions and generative schemes for being and perceiving (Bourdieu 1977, 1990). Bourdieu argues that social history and culture, acquired through the process of socialization, are objectified in habitus, which is the source of an individual's way of being and perceiving. Of paramount importance to the concept of habitus, and of relevance to my analysis here, is that the power of habitus derives from the nonconsciousness of habituation rather than consciously learned principles and rules (Bourdieu 1990). In this sense, music making and music appreciation remain intact because dispositions and forms of know-how are internalized, function below the threshold of cognition, and are enacted as practical sense at a prereflective level. Just as dispositions are embodied and materialized in practice, so is selfhood embodied and manifests in socioculturally specific ways of being-in-the-world (Kontos 2004a).

Wacquant (1992), perhaps Bourdieu's best commentator, notes that Bourdieu is clearly drawing on Merleau-Ponty's idea of the body as the source of practical intentionality and of intersubjective meaning grounded in a preobjective level of experience. The body is treated as a "generative, creative capacity to understand"—as a kind of corporeal awareness—as a practical reason, with reason existing primarily in corporeal ways. With the concept of *habitus*, Bourdieu investigates practice in the context of the social genesis of its conditions of operation. Thus, Bourdieu's exploration of competence, know-how, skill, and disposition leads him into the sociocultural domain in which bodies assume their significance.

One is not born with sociocultural bodily dispositions, but acquires them "by the childhood learning that treats the body as a living memory pad" (Bourdieu 1990, 68). Henry's scat performance demonstrates a cultural aspect of his embodied selfhood determined by his cultural heritage. Thus, determinations attached to primary socialization and one's cultural environment give selfhood its sociocultural specificity by virtue of being embodied and materialized in habitual states, tendencies, and, in the case of Henry, in culturally distinct styles of music. Ritualized patterns of action render cultural possibilities embodied inevitabilities (Bowman 2004). Similarly Malcolm's free jazz performance was consistent with his experience with improvisation and composition of modern jazz, and avant-garde trends (Pickles and Jones 2006). That socially and culturally distinct dimensions of musicality are visibly manifest despite impaired cognition attests to Bourdieu's argument that sociocultural dispositions are regulated not by any conscious obeisance to external rules but by the taken-for-granted, prereflective nature of habitus.

Henry's Calloway-style scat talking and Malcolm's impromptu free jazz performance further resonate with Bourdieu's argument that habitus should be understood not as mechanically constraining action but rather as permitting an element of inventiveness and creativity, albeit within the limits of its structures, which are the embodied sedimentations of the social structures that produced it. Habitus is "a generative spontaneity which asserts itself in the improvised confrontation with endlessly renewed situations," and it "follows a *practical logic*, that of the fuzzy, of the more-or-less, which defines the ordinary relating to the world" (Wacquant 1992, 22). It is this fuzzy and vague but no less masterful capacity to relate to the world that makes it possible for Henry and Malcolm to express themselves in such highly improvisatory music traditions as sound poetry in African-American music and modern jazz, respectively. I argue that these examples render visible how selfhood emanates from the body as a generative spontaneity that asserts itself in an improvised engagement with the world.

Conclusion

In the documentary film, *Alive Inside*, Oliver Sacks, whose case studies of neurological anomalies underscore essential characteristics of the imagination, says "music imprints itself on the brain deeper than any other human experience" and thus just as with other forms of creativity, such as painting

(Kontos 2012, 2003), it is for Sacks "the deepest part of one's being, and may be preserved, almost to the last, in a dementia" (quoted in Storr 1995, 51). However, rather than seeing Henry's resurgence as a testimony to the potential of the human brain, I have argued that the continued implementation of musical intention in the face of neurological impairment is a testimony to the primordial and sociocultural sources of embodied selfhood. This suggests a depth that goes beyond inscription on the brain to a *prereflective* mastery of the world by way of immersion within it. As such the cases of Henry and Malcolm invite a rethinking of conventional notions of music perception, calling for the understanding of such creativity not as the exclusive privilege of the sphere of conscious will but also emanating from our corporeal depths. It entails a shift in the current preoccupation with musical cognition to musical embodiment.

Thinking of selfhood as embodied offers a critical approach to the body that invites a carefully contextualized discussion and exploration of the localized symbiosis of prereflective intentionality and structures of the social world. It is a symbiosis that is "enacted at every instant in the movement of existence" (Merleau-Ponty 1962, 89) rendering the animated, living, experiential body of paramount importance for understanding musical embodiment, selfhood, and dementia. Henry and Malcolm stand as a refutation of closure and an affirmation of discovery and ingenuity. Beyond that, their musicality, as I have argued, is also a powerful reminder that the intelligibility of the body is primary to the continuity of our being.

Acknowledgments

I am presently supported by a Canadian Institutes of Health Research New Investigator Award (MSH-87726, 2009–2014), which facilitated the writing of this chapter. I also acknowledge the support of the Toronto Rehabilitation Institute-University Health Network, which receives funding under the Provincial Rehabilitation Research Program from the Ministry of Health and Long-Term Care in Ontario. The views expressed do not necessarily reflect those of Canadian Institutes of Health Research or the Ministry.

Note

1. My emphasis on an essential corporeality of the self that is separate from cognition does suggest a dualism; however, the focus of my critique is not dualism per se but rather Cartesianism. Contra Cartesianism, the perspective I advance recognizes properties of the body that are essential to selfhood without denying the significance of cognition.

References

Aristotle. 1991. *De Anima*. Translated by R. D. Hicks. Buffalo: Prometheus Books.
Bourdieu, Pierre. 1977. *Outline of a Theory of Practice*. Translated by R. Nice. Cambridge: Cambridge University Press.
———. 1984. *Distinction: A Social Critique of the Judgement of Taste*. Translated by Richard Nice. Cambridge, MA: Harvard University Press.
———. 1990. *The Logic of Practice*. Translated by R. Nice. Cambridge: Polity Press.
Bowman, Wayne D. 1998. *Philosophical Perspectives on Music*. New York: Oxford University Press.
———. 2004. "Cognition and the Body: Perspectives from Music Education." In *Knowing Bodies, Moving Minds: Toward Embodied Teaching and Learning*, edited by Liora Bresler. Netherlands: Kluwer Academic Press.
Bowman, Wayne D., and Kimberly Powell. 2007. "The Body in a State of Music." In *International Handbook of Research in Arts Education*, edited by Liora Bresler. Dordrecht, Netherlands: Springer.
Cohen, Donna, and Carl Eisdorfer. 1986. *The Loss of Self: A Family Resource for the Care of Alzheimer's Disease and Related Disorders*. London: W.W. Norton.
Cuddy, Lola L., and Jacalyn M. Duffin. 2005. "Music, Memory, and Alzheimer's Disease: Is Music Recognition Spared in Dementia, and How Can it be Assessed?" *Medical Hypotheses* 64: 229–235.
Davis, Daniel. 2004. "Dementia: Sociological and Philosophical Constructions." *Social Science and Medicine* 58 (2): 369–378.
Elliott, David. 1991. "Music as knowledge." *Journal of Aesthetic Education* 25 (3): 21–40.
Fontana, Andrea, and Ronald W. Smith. 1989. "Alzheimer's Disease Victims: The 'Unbecoming' of Self and the Normalization of Competence." *Sociological Perspectives* 32 (1): 35–46.
Gibbs, Raymond W. 2005. *Embodiment and Cognitive Science*. Cambridge: Cambridge University Press.
Herskovitz, Elizabeth. 1995. "Struggling over Subjectivity: Debates about the 'Self' and Alzheimer's Disease." *Medical Anthropology Quarterly* 9 (2): 146–164.
Holgersen, Sven-Erik. 2010. "Body Consciousness and Somaesthetics in Music Education." *Action, Criticism, and Theory for Music Education* 9 (1): 31–44.
Juslin, Patrik N., and John A. Sloboda, editors. 2001. *Music and Emotion*. Oxford: Oxford University Press.
Kitwood, Tom, and Kathleen Bredin. 1992. "Towards a Theory of Dementia Care: Personhood and Well-being." *Ageing and Society* 12: 269–287.
Kontos, Pia. 2003. "'The Painterly Hand': Embodied Consciousness and Alzheimer's Disease." *Journal of Aging Studies* 17: 151–170.
———. 2004a. "Ethnographic Reflections on Selfhood, Embodiment and Alzheimer's Disease." *Ageing and Society* 24: 829–849.
———. 2004b. "Local Biology: Reclaiming Body Matter." *Philosophy in the Contemporary World* 11 (Special Issue 1): 87–93.
———. 2005. "Embodied Selfhood in Alzheimer's Disease: Rethinking Person-centred Care." *Dementia: The International Journal of Social Research and Practice* 4 (4): 553–570.
———. 2006. "Embodied Selfhood: An Ethnographic Exploration of Alzheimer's Disease." In *Thinking About Dementia: Culture, Loss, and the Anthropology of Senility*, edited by Lawrence Cohen and Annette Leibing. New Brunswick, NJ: Rutgers University Press.
———. 2012. "Alzheimer's Expressions or Expressions Despite Alzheimer's? Philosophical Reflections on Self and Embodiment." *Occasion: Interdisciplinary Studies in the Humanities* 4: 1–12.
Kontos, Pia, Karen-Lee Miller, and Gail J. Mitchell. 2010. "Neglecting the Importance of the Decision Making and Care Regimes of Personal Support Workers: A Critique of Standardization of Care Planning Through the RAI/MDS." *The Gerontologist* 50 (3): 352–362.

Kontos, Pia, Gail J. Mitchell, Bahvnita Mistry, and Bruce Ballon. 2010. "Using Drama to Improve Person-centred Dementia Care." *International Journal of Older People Nursing* 5: 159–168.

Kontos, Pia, and Gary Naglie. 2007a. "Bridging Theory and Practice: Imagination, the Body, and Person-centred Dementia Care." *Dementia: The International Journal of Social Research and Practice* 6 (4): 549–569.

———. 2007b. "'Expressions of Personhood in Alzheimer's Disease': An Evaluation of Research-based Theatre as a Pedagogical Tool." *Qualitative Health Research* 17 (6): 799–811.

Matthews, Eric. 2006. "Dementia and the Identity of the Person." In *Dementia: Mind, Meaning and the Person*, edited by Jilian C. Hughes, Stephen J. Louw, and Steven R. Sabat. Oxford: Oxford University Press.

Maus, Fred E. 2010. "Somaesthetics of Music." *Action, Criticism, and Theory for Music Education* 9 (1): 9–25.

Merleau-Ponty, Maurice. 1962. *Phenomenology of Perception*. Translated by C. Smith. London: Routledge & K. Paul.

———. 1964. "An Unpublished Text by Maurice Merleau-Ponty: A Prospectus of his Work." In *The Primacy of Perception*, edited by James Edie. Evanston: Northwestern University Press.

Ortega, Francisco. 2009. "The Cerebral Subject and the Challenge of Neurodiversity." *BioSocieties* 4: 425–445.

Pickles, Vernon, and Raya A. Jones. 2006. "The Persons Still Comes First: The Continuing Musical Self in Dementia." *Journal of Consciousness Studies* 13 (3): 73–93.

Ronch, Judah L. 1996. "Mourning and Grief in Late Life Alzheimer's Dementia: Revisiting the Vanishing Self." *American Journal of Alzheimer's Disease* 11 (4): 25–28.

Rossato-Bennett, Michael. 2012. Alive Inside [Film], accessed December 6, 2012, http://www.youtube.com/watch?v=fyZQf0p73QM&list=UUWSW0VyPUvG8dfJc9VtFQRg&index=3&feature=plcp.

Shusterman, Richard. 2010. "Body Consciousness and Music: Variations on Some Themes." *Action, Criticism, and Theory for Music Education* 9 (1): 1–23.

Storr, Rovert. 1995. "'At Last Light.'" In *Willem de Kooning: The Late Paintings, The 1980s*, edited by Janet Jenkins. Minneapolis, MN: Walker Art Center and San Francisco Museum of Modern Art.

Vidal, Fernando. 2009. "Brainhood, Anthropological Figure of Modernity." *History of the Human Sciences* 22 (1): 5–36.

Wacquant, Loïc J. D. 1992. "Toward a Social Praxeology: The Structure and Logic of Bourdieu's Sociology." In *An Invitation to Reflexive Sociology*, edited by Pierre Bourdieu and Loïc Wacquant, 2–59. Chicago: University of Chicago Press.

Watson, P. 1999. Alzheimer's: A True Story [Film], accessed December 6, 2012, http://digital.films.com/play/KUG6RA.

8

As the Body Speaks: Creative Expression in Dementia

ALISON PHINNEY

Coming to Dementia

As a nurse who works with older people, my interest in the study of dementia has been with me for a long time. I often trace it back to an opportunity I had as a young psychology student to conduct neuropsychological testing with adults who had been diagnosed as children with significant learning disabilities. I remember two young men in particular, neither one of whom was able to read with any degree of fluency. One was doing well in his life, happily moving forward in a successful business career, while the other was working as a custodian at a fast food restaurant and pleaded with me to help him learn to read. While their specific disabilities were remarkably similar, I was struck by how different their lives were and wondered how this could be. Ultimately, it was this curiosity that led me to the study and eventual practice of nursing, where I felt I could best find comfortable middle ground between what I understood as the physical (in this case, neurological impairment) and the human aspects of what I might now call "lived experience."

Some years later, working in a psychiatric hospital in Montreal, I had my first real encounter with dementia. In these years and in this place, we talked about "organic brain syndrome." I had read about this as a student, and had taken a course in neuroanatomy with the remarkable James Brawer at McGill University, so I understood something about the brain structures that were affected and how memory and eventually language and mobility could all be lost. But understanding this did little to support my everyday practice as a nurse caring for older people who walked the hallways day after day, unsure of where they were, who seemed to recognize me but could not remember my name, and who enjoyed listening to music but had no words to share their experience. Mostly I was curious, wondering what it was like to live with this disease.

I carried that curiosity with me as I found my way back to the research world. The timing was right to be asking this question. Pharmaceutical companies were looking for people with early dementia to test the new drugs that were just coming to market, which had the effect of creating a certain kind of "subject pool" of people who were willing and able to take part in a study that asked them about their experiences living with this disease. At the same time, scholars were starting to talk about personhood and identity in dementia. Steve Sabat in the United States and Tom Kitwood in the United Kingdom had each in their own way drawn attention to the problematic discourse around the self in dementia, challenging societal assumptions that through loss of memory and language people become less than fully human (Kitwood 1990; Sabat and Harré 1992). These two things happening together shifted the ground a bit, opening up possibilities for new ways of thinking about and doing research with dementia.

My earliest work came quite naturally from the questions that had emerged from my practice as a nurse. How do people living with dementia experience and make sense of their symptoms? This is a good nursing question, trying as it does to dwell in that middle ground between biomedicine (talking of symptoms of disease) and the human sciences (talking of lived experience and meaning). In this chapter, I begin by laying out some of the conceptual thinking that characterizes that middle ground, ultimately foregrounding the place of the lived body in everyday experience. My most recent work has been exploring so-called meaningful activity in dementia, and in this chapter I focus specifically on people's involvement in the creative arts as an exemplar of how experience is expressed and understood through the lived body.

Conceptual Traditions

Raising the idea of middle ground is admittedly problematic. It is an inherently dualist metaphor, and it was the problems I perceived with dualist thinking that got me started on this journey in the first place. The Lockean notion that the person is a self-contained entity consisting of determinate properties (e.g. cognitive capacity, affective state, or behavioral condition) living in but separate from the environment, seemed to me to be wrong somehow. As a nurse, I resisted being backed into a corner, forced to focus on the loss of the very properties that are deemed essential to personhood. Nor was I comfortable with the assumption that the world exists as an objective entity beyond ourselves and that we rely on our perceptual and cognitive abilities to see and understand this external world. It seemed to lead all too easily to the inevitable conclusion that people with dementia become alienated from the world and others around them.

Such assumptions have contributed to a research model that excludes the person's experience as a source of understanding and meaning. Instead, their experience living with dementia is considered to be both idiosyncratic and inaccessible. Furthermore, the model is based on the belief that the person's capacity to self-interpret is impaired. Their perspective on their own experience is viewed with suspicion, assumed to be fundamentally flawed, based on misperceptions and misunderstandings.

Through the past decade, these kinds of assumptions have to some extent gone by the wayside. The growing body of "subjective experience" literature demonstrates that people with dementia are able to reflect on their experiences and share their perceptions with others and the question of "accuracy" has been largely dismissed, courtesy in part of prevailing postmodern views of the person with dementia as the expert in their own private experience and concepts of reality as fundamentally subjective. Thus, that particular species of dualism is perhaps not as relevant a critique at this point in time. Kitwood's view of personhood in dementia as socially constructed has gained considerable traction (1997), which would seem to have found some way at least around the problematic subject-object divide.

However, as human beings we seem inevitably drawn to lines of division, and I would argue that much of the rhetoric around personhood and identity in dementia continues to be caught up in dualist thinking. The desire to make dementia care better has drawn scholars together and everyone agrees with the moral imperative of seeing the patient as a person. However, the fact that we are embodied persons has never really found a place in the discussion. No one denies the fact of dementia as a brain disease, but considerable effort over the past two decades has gone toward articulating a social science perspective that will somehow act as a corrective to what is perceived as the "biomedicalization" of dementia (Lyman 1989). The biological has been relegated to the margins of this discourse around personhood, self, and identity, with the resulting effect that the lived body has been largely ignored as a conceptual category.

Coming to the Body

As a nurse, this puts me in a difficult "either-or" kind of place. This view of body and person as conceptually distinct sets up difficult tensions that have led me to consider alternative perspectives; in what follows, I lay out some of the concepts that are most important to my work, presenting these as the tools I use to negotiate a way through this landscape.

To begin with, it has always been important to me that I be able to attend to the context of people's lives, taking account of the significance or *meaning* of their situation, which is shaped by their history and their day-to-day experiences. It was this that caught my attention all those years ago when I met those two young men who could not read, and it continues to be this same issue now in my work in the area of dementia.

A view of meaning as that which is disclosed in and through experience living in the world is something I arrived at in part through a reading of Heidegger, and in particular his idea of "being-in-the-world." With this language, Heidegger (1962) is discarding the traditional subject-object distinction, being careful to point out that "subject and Object do not coincide with *Dasein* and the world" (87). Instead, *Dasein* is constituted by *being-in-the-world*, which may be best understood in terms of our everyday familiarity and involved practical dealings that disclose the world as intelligible to us.

Merleau-Ponty further developed these ideas, speaking of how "the world is not what I think but what I live through" (1962, xvi–xvii), and later describing how we experience our perceptions not by explicitly "knowing them," but rather we experience them "in action" "in the world," (Merleau-Ponty 1964, 12). A similar kind of idea was expressed by John Dewey in his book *Art as Experience*, where he explained how experience, "instead of signifying being shut up within one's own private feelings and sensations,... signifies active and alert commerce with the world" (1934, 18).

Heidegger, Merleau-Ponty, and Dewey are all in their own ways pointing to action or practices as foundational to meaning. The point here is that we are not subjects with private inner experiences, but rather it is what we *do* that constitutes meaning. This idea has been influential in my work, leading me to focus on the question of activity, and it was thinking about action and practices that first lead me to consider the importance of the body.

Merleau-Ponty argued that it is not through "intellectual interpretation" but rather "through my body that I understand other people, just as it is through my body that I perceive things" (1962, 185–186). This is the body that I am interested in—not the mechanistic body of Cartesian dualism that operates under direction of causal influences, but rather the body that makes possible our understanding as active involvement in the world (Leonard 1989). It is a situated embodied understanding that allows us to grasp and cope with our environment and with others, and it is this idea that provides the conceptual grounding for the following exploration of experiences of creative activity by people with dementia.

Creative Activity in Dementia

Over the past ten years I have conducted four studies focusing on various aspects of everyday life and activity in dementia. The study participants have been people with Alzheimer's disease or a related dementia (forty-five in total), most of whom were living at home with at least one family member. They represented a range of cognitive impairment. People were between six months and four years postdiagnosis, and typically had some trouble recalling major aspects of their recent experiences and needed varying degrees of help with their daily activities. Most were able to engage reasonably well in a conversation, although a few had considerable trouble using language and relied fairly heavily on family members and/or nonverbal communication. People ranged in age from forty-six to ninety years old, and there were roughly equal numbers of men and women.

In all of this research, our purpose has been to understand people's experience in the context of their everyday lives. We have drawn on methods of ethnographic fieldwork, conducting conversational-style interviews and participant observation with people with dementia and their families in their homes, and gathering video and photographic recordings of their activities. We came to know most people very well, typically meeting with them on four to eight occasions over a period of six to eighteen months.

This research has been focused quite broadly on activity as a general category. Although issues around people's involvement in the arts had been a common thread, it had never been examined on its own terms. Looking more carefully across the data from the four studies, it became apparent that there were seven people who identified themselves as artists, either as professionals or as active amateurs, and that they had much to say about the significance of creative activity in their lives. What follows is an analysis of the data from those seven cases.

Using methods of interpretive phenomenology (Benner 1994), this analysis began with an in-depth read of the data for each person, focusing on their involvement in the arts, and then moving on to explore the contrasts and commonalities across the seven people.

Creative activity is a large domain of potential inquiry. The focus here was on the practices themselves rather than the end products, which is to say the *doing* and *undergoing* of experience (Dewey 1934). The analysis therefore was oriented around three lines of inquiry: (1) What is it that solicits people's involvement in

Table 8.1. **Study participants**

Bob (84 yrs)	Professional musician, choir conductor
Joe (82 yrs)	Amateur musician, harmonica
Don (80 yrs)	Amateur musician, choral singer
Betty (46 yrs)	Professional artist, traditional crafts
Abigail (82 yrs)	Professional artist, watercolor and fiber art
Jim (55 yrs)	Professional artist, ink and pencil drawing
Maxwell (67 yrs)	Amateur artist, pastel paintings

creative activity? (2) What are people's experiences as they carry through with the practice? (3) What does their involvement in creative activity mean to them?

Getting Started

As we spent time with people, it became apparent that although most were doing less than before, they still found ways to engage in creative activity. For this reason, it became important to understand what it was that allowed them to *get started*. The following discussion explores how people *feel the urge* to make art as a kind of sensory experience, but more and more as this urge was fading, they were coming to *rely on the world* around them to provide opportunity and encouragement.

FEELING THE URGE

Getting started begins with how people are feeling, and by that I am referring to the sensory experiences that seemed to draw people forward, or alternatively, that were holding them back from engaging in their art. The example of Betty is one that illustrates how the creative act is at its core a bodily experience. Betty was a woman of aboriginal descent who with the onset of her dementia had experienced what she felt as a kind of creative awakening. She started a business designing native crafts and making "kits" that she parceled out to her employees who in turn manufactured the items and helped sell them at local craft fairs and farmer's markets. But what got all this started and what keeps it going is her creative vision that she experiences as images in her head that are provided to her by her ancestors. She sees an object—a traditional dreamcatcher,[1] a leather bootie for a child, or a necklace—"as clearly as I'm looking at you" she said, and she feels driven to bring these images to life through her creative work.

We spent time with Betty in her workshop as she carefully worked on a beaded necklace, speaking quietly every now and again to explain what compels her to create. "I see the finished product in my head already" she said. "It's being given to me."

This is not a mere intellectual exercise for Betty, turning an image into an object. Rather, her experience is one that is deeply embodied. She sees visual forms that have emerged from within her own being and she has a deep kind of sensory engagement with the objects in her world. Before sitting down to work, she showed the research assistant around the workshop, inviting her to see and touch the tender pieces of leather and soft furs, the colorful feathers and textured beads. It is these experiences of the sensing body-in-the-world that lead her to create.

It was similar for Joe, who as a harmonica player had a "regular gig" at a local community center where he performed every Thursday. Being in an auditorium with other musicians in front of a crowd of people was a familiar way of being-in-the-world for Joe that solicited his performance. Upon hearing the opening strains of a familiar melody, it was a completely natural thing for him to step in close toward the microphone, lift the harmonica to his mouth, and begin to play.

Others were coming to feel this urge less strongly. They spoke of how they were less active, describing this as being "in a lull" or a "slow period." Abigail, for example, had been working for some time on a watercolor, but felt in herself a real sense of inertia, speaking often of how she did not have the energy she had once had. During one of our visits, we watched as she developed the outlines of a waterfront scene from a nearby marina. She sat heavily in her chair, and while she was attentive to the canvas, her movements were minimal and slow. She felt this to be in marked contrast to her level of activity in the past, as evidenced by the paintings, textiles, and sculptures that filled her small apartment to overflowing.

RELYING ON THE WORLD

As people were feeling less drawn toward creative expression, the situations in which they found themselves took on ever more significance. Increasingly, they needed to have the right kind of opportunity and encouragement to get started.

In some cases, they were able to create these opportunities for themselves. For example, Abigail left her art supplies out on the table because if they were out of her sight, her painting would simply not happen. She explained:

> I have this set up for fooling around and doing things. I can use a piece of paper and my paints and my brushes, and they're all there, I don't ever put them away. It's all ready. I think the most horrible thing is to feel like doing something and then having to go get it out because you usually say "Oh well, tomorrow."

Abigail had learned that having the equipment ready made it easier to get started, and in this way, was creating for herself an environment that better afforded her involvement. Others were more reliant on family and friends. Maxwell was an accomplished pastel artist who had slowed to a point where he was making little progress, working just a few hours a week on one small drawing. His wife, also an artist, told us how she liked to "encourage him to do more," offering every now and then a gentle suggestion to work a bit on his art. Sometimes she would bring out her own canvas to work beside him as a way to keep him engaged.

We noticed that the research itself sometimes played a similar role. Jim had done very little drawing since the onset of his dementia, but when we asked about the paintings on the walls of his small apartment, he was led to reflect on his experiences as an artist. This in itself seemed to get him moving again, picking up his sketchpad and trying things out that he could show us at the next visit.

Beyond offering reminders and prompts, family and friends also took it upon themselves to create situations where people were more likely to feel the urge to express themselves creatively. Don had been a talented choral singer since childhood, but as his dementia advanced he had found it impossible to keep up with the group. Understanding the importance of music in his life, Don's wife had arranged for members of the choir to visit on a regular basis to play the piano and sing with him. We had the chance to witness this, being there on a day when a friend was scheduled to come by. Don seemed frail and disengaged; there was a kind of precariousness and uncertainty in his demeanor as he sat waiting, perched on the arm of an easy chair. However, when his friend sat next to him at the piano and started to play, Don immediately burst into song with a voice that was deep and strong and confident. This was a man who could describe with great eloquence how important singing was to him, but his actual involvement was only possible because others had created a world for him that allowed that desire to speak itself, almost as if a switch had been turned on.

Carrying Through

The idea of *carrying through* is used in reference to people's experiences of "doing and undergoing" creative activity. For some, their experience was one of *smooth flow*, of being caught up in activity that seemed to carry them along with little effort on their part. But more and more, carrying through was characterized by a sense of breakdown that served to *interrupt* the creative act.

SMOOTH FLOW

The paradigm case for me of artistic performance as embodied smooth flow has long been the story of Bob, one of the very first participants in my research. Bob was a retired choral conductor who had recently had an opportunity to perform at a college reunion. He shared with me the video recording of the concert and I was struck by how different he seemed once he stepped up on the podium. Bob shuffled slowly across the stage, his shoulders bent and his gaze cast down, but as the performance began, he stood tall, rarely looking to the score, moving his entire body with the music as he motioned to the different sections, never missing an entrance. After showing me the video, he spoke of how pleased he had been with this performance, taking great effort to explain how it was a matter of expressing the music through his body.

> 'When you are conducting a choral group, it isn't a matter of beating time, but of expressing what it is.... Everything they sing, I do here.' There is a sense in which it just 'comes out' without any thought or effort on his part. He explained: 'My arms to this day, can just conduct. Fly away.' It has become for him effortless and transparent, in his words 'just so very, very easy. When it works, it is just great!' (Phinney, 2011, 259)

Although Bob is the person who expressed it best of all these artists, there are others who have similar experiences. Joe's wife explained that once he gets going, he will not want to stop, and we saw this too. When he stepped onto the stage at the community center, once he began playing it seemed effortless, as if the music itself was carrying him through.

Abigail, in reflecting on her experience of painting, described a similar kind of bodily engagement that happened as she became caught up in creative activity. Putting the pencil to paper was still very easy she explained. Sketching out the preliminary ideas was something that was quite "unconscious"; the lines just happened. While she had less energy to start painting, once she put the brush to canvas, it felt little different from before. "The hand, the eye, it's just the same, it's better."

INTERRUPTION

For many of these artists, however, this experience of embodied smooth flow was beginning to diminish. Abigail herself felt more often forced to stop and reflect on what she has done, to consider the composition for example, or the way the colors were working together. We saw this as we watched her at work. There were brief moments of activity, followed by long pauses when she held the brush to the side, shifting her gaze back and forth across the painting, looking to the pallet and back again. She explained to us later that in the past there had been fewer of these interrupted moments, mostly because she had been able to work more quickly. Now it took her longer to figure out what was working in the painting and what was not, and to decide what she might do to fix it.

This kind of interruption was apparent for others as well. When Don was singing, he would often forget the words and the music would falter, but his wife and his friends had quickly become adept at cueing him with the next line just before it was needed. He would hear these words and most of the time was able to take them up so the song could go on with minimal interruption.

For others, the interruption was irreparable. Jim's efforts to draw were a paradigm case of this kind of breakdown. His language was failing him, but through words and gesture he reflected on how he was trying to draw more, but was finding it challenging. He might start a sketch, but something in the world would move he said, and the moment was gone. He could not recapture it and the drawing was left unfinished. He shared with us fragmented sketches of a piece of driftwood lying on the beach. The lines were faint and incomplete, offering the barest hint of the dried twisted roots of an old cedar tree.

Jim clearly conveyed his frustration at being interrupted in this way, shaking his head and clenching his fist as he spoke. This was a man whose practice as an artist was very diminished, although he continued to approach the world with an artist's eye. He spent many hours every day walking through his neighborhood, watching people and places with a particular intensity, and yet his ability to make ready sense of this world and to bring that understanding to life through his drawing was starting to break down. His faltering description of how "the world moves" and the moment is gone is evocative, leading one to consider how experiences of interruption are a kind of disruption of body-world integration.

Meaning

These seven artists were different in terms of what kind of art they practiced, how long they had been doing it, and to what extent it had provided for them a living. But all of them shared the feeling that this was a most significant part of their lives and they wanted us to understand how much it mattered to them. This question of meaning is not a straightforward story; the importance of creative expression is, in the words of one of the participants, "a multifaceted kind of thing."

CONTINUITY

One facet is almost certainly something to do with identity and the self. In previous work I have described how people through involvement in activity continue to live up to the demands of previous work identities, for example Bob, who continued to embody his role as a professional musician. The practices of a conductor still came to him easily, and the smooth-flowing unencumbered performance is one that felt to Bob the same as ever. The music resided "deep inside" he explained, and was untouched by the dementia. He *felt* himself to be the same person he had always been (Phinney, Chaudhury, and O'Connor 2007).

This sense of continuity over time and place was something we heard from those participants who shared with us how their art was something that had been with them for many years. Don told the story of how he had started singing as a very young boy, first at school and then later in community choruses and how it had continued throughout his adult years. As he said "[music] has been one ongoing part of my, of what I, [it's] sort of who I am.... once you get into a skill, a habit, a natural urge to do music, it soon comes a part of who you are and what you understand." In these words we hear Don explaining how music is for him an embodied capacity that has built up over time, allowing him to express who he is. Having seen him sing together with his friend at the piano, we too understood how through his performance of traditional Christian hymns, he was able once again to inhabit his role as a church leader.

It was similar for Joe who continues to play the traditional music he learned as a young boy. According to his wife, Joe has always "related" to the east coast of Canada where he grew up, but it is an even stronger feeling now. Every night before he goes to sleep, he imagines the small fishing village of his childhood, and especially when he plays the music, he is filled with a sense of unbroken connection with his past.

CONNECTION

Time and again in our interviews, people talked about the deep feelings of happiness and satisfaction they experienced by doing their art for and with others. This relational aspect of creative activity is easy to see in the case of the musicians because the performance aspect is integral and immediate, but it was also true for the visual artists. Maxwell discovered that people really liked his work and he could sell his drawings. He spoke frankly about there being two reasons why his art was important to him: not only did he find pleasure in the creative act itself—what he described as "painting for the sheer joy of painting"—but even more when the resulting product was enjoyed by someone else. "It's creating something that other people will derive pleasure from," he said.

While Joe said he sometimes liked to play when he was at home by himself, mostly his music was about his relationships with others, and his wife especially. At every interview, there would come a time toward the end when he would pick up his harmonica and play her a love song, watching her intently as he played, never breaking eye contact. He did this at the community center too. She explained: "He does a nice thing for me. He stands at the mike and I know when he points at me that he is going to play one for me and he says 'This one is for Louise' and he plays 'Have I told You Lately that I Love You.'" It was important to Joe to see people enjoying his music. When we watched him play at the community center, there was something quite unique in how he held himself. While the other musicians held their heads low toward their instruments, or looked to each other as they played, Joe never stopped watching the audience. When asked later what it was like to play there each week he answered: "I can get a feeling I'm looking at the crowd, I can look right at them.... They're singing it. You can see their lips. They're in perfect time with me." For Joe, having an audience was most important. He came to feel a sense of almost bodily connection with others through his music.

Beyond their connection with others, through their involvement in creative activity people also experienced a sense of connection and belonging in the world. As Don explained: "Music is stimulating, it gives you opportunities to participate, in choruses and music groups, and activities that are music inclined, it's just a great way to take part in the life of the city." It was for this reason perhaps that he had recently taken up dancing at the local community center. Although he could no longer manage the demands of being a choir member, his body could still execute a fox trot or a waltz, and it was a joy to him to be dancing with others as the music played.

Betty's experience was very much about how through her art she has finally found a sense of belonging and connection with her aboriginal heritage. She talked about how she had been alienated from this community as a young child. "When I was a kid it was a bad thing to talk about the native in us. So it was always put away. You never talked about it. You never discussed it." When she discovered she had dementia, she was left with a sense of limited time and decided that she had to learn as much as she could about her background. She told the story of what happened next.

> And then, one day a friend said 'Could you help me clean the craft room?' and she came up with a feather and some leather. And I saw this really strong vision in my head. And I thought 'I'm going to make this,' and I did. I strongly feel that what's happening with me on this business is that my ancestors are pushing me to make the stuff, because the visions are so strong.

It is as if through her body she is bringing the world of her ancestors into existence, incorporating literally her native heritage through her craft.

DELIGHT

In the past I have written about how activity can be meaningful to the extent that it brings people pleasure and enjoyment (Phinney, Chaudhury, and O'Connor 2007). I have tended to think of this as an obvious and not terribly important finding, choosing to pay attention to the more weighty matters of significance—people's sense of purpose, or matters of identity. But listening to artists talk about their activity makes it very clear that these feelings were what mattered most. People fumbled for words, but did their best to convey about just how good it feels to be sketching the outlines of a boat, playing a well-loved song, or designing a traditional mask: "It feels great"; "There is no better feeling"; "It feels so good." We heard these words again and again, and we saw it too. In Joe's performance at the community center, he swayed in time to the music and finished with a joyful flourish, his arm raised in celebration.

Don, as a retired minister, was the most eloquent in describing this sense of deep and abiding delight. Music he said "fills up my interest, my activities, my time, my desire..." Later he went on to say:

> To put it very bluntly, singing is just a blessing I think. A blessing...that I can express joy and happiness and all the good things that come with it, and fun, and the expression, and all the dynamics that goes with music and what you can do with music...I think it's just one of the most wonderful things that god created for us. I don't know how I can say it better.

This perhaps speaks to the idea of delight not as a separate "category" of meaning to be considered in addition to the idea of artistic performance as embodying identity or forging connection with the broader world, but rather as the emotional experience that binds all these "facets" together. It is the feeling that creates the possibility for activity to be meaningful at all.

These emotional experiences seemed to be the most important thread throughout these studies, being revealing both in the interviews and the observations, but by their very nature they are hard to thematize. These are feelings of the body, the body speaking as it were, and there are perhaps no words.

Final Thoughts

In this chapter I have examined experiences of artists with dementia in an effort to understand the significance of creative activity by directing attention to the body that "carries forth" the meaning of a situation (Johnson 2007). The analysis has brought to light two important qualities of this situated embodied understanding.

First, it has uncovered how the *engaged body* that negotiates surroundings and interacts with objects is being transformed. Although people might still find themselves fully absorbed in creative expression, enjoying the smooth flow of their "ready-to-hand" involvement (Heidegger 1962), this was happening less often. Moments of interruption were becoming more frequent, leaving them with a sense of being detached from the world.

Second, people's experience of creative expression is revealing of how the *sensing body* exists as the "feeling of what happens" (Damasio 1999). Although their situations varied, what was held in common by all the participants were the very powerful feelings engendered through their engagement in creative activities. It is this "embodied *felt* experience [that] is expressed in the art itself" (Cresswell and Baerveldt 2011, 266), whether it be a musical performance, a painting, or a traditional craft. At the same time, however, the urge to make art is fading as the body weakens and becomes less active.

In summary, for these artists with dementia, creative expression occurs in and through the body that carries through activity even while it is faltering, that retains the capacity for delight even while the desire to create is diminished. The body is telling of both possibilities; it cannot be one or the other. Rather, theirs is an experience of being betwixt and between, dwelling in a kind of liminal space that is at once beyond and in the midst of loss.

And the tree was happy.
— Shel Silverstein, *The Giving Tree*, 1964

Note

1. In the North American indigenous tradition, a dreamcatcher is a webbed hoop decorated with beads and feathers. It is considered to carry both personal and sacred significance.

References

Benner, Patricia. 1994. *Interpretive Phenomenology: Embodiment, Caring and Ethics in Health and Illness*. Thousand Oaks, CA: Sage Publications.
Cresswell, J., and C. Baerveldt. 2011. Bakhtin's Realism and Embodiment: Toward a Revision of the Dialogical Self. *Culture and Psychology* 17: 263–277.
Damasio, Antonio. 1999. *The Feeling of What Happens: Body and Emotion in the Making of Consciousness*. London: Heinneman.
Dewey, John. 1934. *Art as Experience*. New York: Penguin.
Heidegger, Martin. 1962. *Being and Time*. Translated by John Macquarrie and Edward Robinson. London: SCM Press.
Johnson, Mark. 2007. *The Meaning of the Body: Aesthetics of Human Understanding*. Chicago: University of Chicago Press.
Kitwood, Tom. 1990. "The Dialectics of Dementia: With Particular Reference to Alzheimer Disease." *Ageing and Society* 10: 177–196.
Kitwood, Tom. 1997. *Dementia Reconsidered: The Person Comes First*. Buckingham: Open University Press.
Leonard, V. W. 1989. "A Heideggerean Phenomenologic Perspective on the Concept of the Person." *Advances in Nursing Science* 11 (4): 40–55.
Lyman, K. 1989. "Bringing the Social Back In: A Critique of the Bio-medicalization of Dementia." *The Gerontologist* 29: 597–605.
Merleau-Ponty, Maurice. 1962. *Phenomenology of Perception*. Translated by Colin Smith. London: Routledge.

———. 1964. "The Primacy of Perception and its Philosophical Consequences." In *The Primacy of Perception*, edited by J. Edie, 12–42. Chicago: Northwestern University Press.

Phinney, Alison. 2011. "Horizons of Meaning in Dementia: Retained and Shifting Narratives." *Journal of Religion, Spirituality and Aging* 23: 254–268.

Phinney, Alison, Habib Chaudhury, and Deborah O'Connor. 2007. "Doing as Much as I Can Do: The Meaning of Activity for People with Dementia." *Aging and Mental Health* 11: 384–393.

Sabat, Steve, and Rom Harré. 1992. "The Construction and Deconstruction of Self in Alzheimer's Disease." *Ageing and Society* 12: 443–461.

Part Three

COMMUNICATION, FAMILY, AND INSTITUTIONS

9

How to Do Things with Others: Joint Activities Involving Persons with Alzheimer's Disease

LARS-CHRISTER HYDÉN

Oswald and Linda have been married for almost fifty years and are, at the time of the interview, around seventy years old. The interview is part of a larger ongoing research project involving joint interviews with ten couples where one spouse has Alzheimer's disease (AD). Oswald has an academic background while Linda has worked as a secretary, and has also taken care of the couple's three children. At the time of the interview Oswald is diagnosed with AD and has cognitive problems, particularly with remembering; he has a limited linguistic register, problems finding words, and also pronunciation problems; he tends to make some syntactic errors (especially verb tense) and is only able to make short contributions—a memory fragment, a phrase or a couple of words, or acknowledge that he hears a contribution. As a consequence, Linda has become extremely important to Oswald. The example below is from the beginning of the interview, when one of the interviewers asked the couple to tell about when they met the first time. (For further information about the example, see Hydén 2011a.)

Early on in the example Oswald signals that he has not grasped the question and he asks a question in order to get a clarification. It takes the couple around fifteen turns just to reach an agreement about the meaning of the initial question that Linda poses: "Where did we meet?"

This example is in many ways typical for conversations involving persons with AD, particularly in its more advanced stages. Both Oswald and Linda spend considerable time in order to understand a fairly small item in the conversation, something that also characterizes the rest of the interview: during the forty-five minutes they take to tell their story they devote at least half of that time to reaching an understanding of what they mean or refer to (see Hydén 2011a).

1	L:	where did we meet?
2	O:	where we met
3	L:	yes
4	O:	met on what
5	L:	first time
6	O:	first time
7	L:	Yes
8	O:	yes ((hesitant))
9		((pause 3 seconds))
10		Yes
11		first time
12		yes yes it must have been whewhewhen iiiit we was when we were newnewnew
13	Both:	((laughter))
14	O:	new new neewl newl
15		what's it called
16	L:	but the first time that we met
17		we were at a party
18	O:	meby so ((maybe so)) yes that was the way it was
19	L:	Yes
20	O:	but then it was
21		then it was like that yes
22		that SOMEONE
23		YOU
24	L:	yes
25	O:	who met someone
26	L:	yes I met YOU then yes
26	O:	yes

Although all persons with AD live with other persons during their illness, very little research has been conducted on *joint activities*—like the conversation in the example—involving persons with AD. Much of the research on AD has focused on describing and explaining the diseased individual's declining cognitive and linguistic abilities. Little research has dealt with the ways persons with AD actually cope with these losses. Even less research has engaged with how persons with AD together with other persons—jointly, as in the example—cope with the potential problems that result from these losses. A theoretical shift away from the individual with AD to a focus on the person with AD as a participant engaged in collaboration with other participants would help to describe and understand how the declining cognitive and linguistic abilities are dealt with jointly. This would be interesting because it could help us conceptualize the consequences of AD less as an individual problem than as something that is dealt with in everyday interaction *together* with other persons. This implies viewing the losses involved in AD as being part of the interactional network of the person with AD and hence as something involving many other persons. A theoretical shift would also imply that we could investigate and describe the ways the participants organize their collaboration in order to deal with the potential problems that may or actually do emerge in the interaction. In general, this is also knowledge with practical implications that could contribute to changing the notion of persons with dementia.

This chapter is about developing a network of concepts for understanding the collaboration between Oswald and Linda, as seen in the previous example. In particular, I want to do two things. First, I suggest that the notion of joint activities can function as a theoretical tool that can be used to describe and discuss the organization of collaboration involving persons with AD. The joint activities progress through new contributions made by the individual participants; the participants must negotiate these contributions in order to establish the meaning of the contribution so the activity can proceed. Second, as the person with AD progressively loses some of the cognitive and linguistic abilities that are important in joint activities, the person without AD has to take on a greater responsibility for the activity. This renegotiated organization of the collaboration can be discussed in terms of the creation of "scaffolds" that both parties can use in order to negotiate shared meaning and hence be able to continue their joint activities. To present the argument I discuss these issues in relation to collaboration between one person with AD and one person without AD—although real life collaborations also may take place between two (or more) persons with AD, or in larger groups involving both person with and without AD.

The chapter continues with a brief review of some of the experimental research on AD and the limitations of the individualistic theories for understanding what persons with AD can and cannot do. This is followed by an overview of the theoretical ideas and conceptions associated with joint activities. Of particular relevance in this context is the fact that joint activities suppose the participants' mutual support, something that is central to research on AD. The rest of the chapter discusses ways to structure and conceptualize the various kinds of problems that emerge in interactions involving persons with AD, and how the participants can deal with these problems.

The Lonely Alzheimer Individual

Much of the research on persons with AD has been based on experimental studies. In these studies the person with AD is facing the experimental tasks on his or her own. Interaction with the researcher is generally neither part of the study design nor noted in the results section. The aim is to study the "internal" cognitive and linguistic abilities and losses as such in "pure form" without interfering influence from various kinds of external factors.

At the same time, the fact that neither the social context, nor the interaction between the person with AD and the experimenter, nor the actual character of the task, are taken into account becomes a problem with most of these experimental studies. Several researchers have found that interaction with others during an experiment or interview actually affects the abilities of the persons with AD and hence what this person is able to accomplish.

In research on storytelling abilities, some investigators have designed interview studies in which persons with AD tell autobiographical stories, often together with a spouse or another significant person (Blonder, Kort, and Schmitt 1994; Hamilton 1994; Ramanathan 1997; Usita, Hyman, and Herman 1998), on the hypothesis that autobiographical storytelling is a more immediately meaningful task as compared to retelling some other kind of story. It is also suggested that the interaction between the storyteller with AD and listeners may be important. In a unique study, Kemper and her colleagues (1995) found that if persons with AD were assigned the task of telling stories together with their spouses, the spouses supported and helped their partners with the task. As a consequence of this the persons with AD were able to tell "significantly longer and more elaborated personal narratives in collaboration with their spouses than they were able to tell in the solo condition" (Kemper, Lyons, and Anagnopoulos 1995, 214). Persons with AD also had fewer word-finding problems during joint storytelling and were better at retrieving missing details in response to their spouses' prompts. The researchers' conclusion is that "patients with AD are able to communicate more effectively with their spouses' help and assistance than they are able to alone. Spouses can provide contextual cues for the participants, settings, and significant events in the lives of the patients with AD" (215).

Surprisingly few studies have continued this line of research; most research still focuses on the storytelling of the isolated individual with AD. What Kemper et al.'s study indicates is that something happens in the interaction between the persons with AD and their spouses that helps the persons with AD become better storytellers, both in terms of the number of words used as well as recalled events. One possible aspect of special interest could be the interactional, compensatory strategies used by the spouses in order to enhance the participation of the person with AD in the storytelling—something not discussed by Kemper and her colleagues.

Reconceptualizing AD and Collaboration

This brief review of previous research strongly suggests that some of the findings from experimental research contradict the individualistic theoretical assumptions and instead indicate that interaction and collaboration are important to better understand persons with AD. This indicates the need for a theoretical framework for describing and understanding joint activities and collaboration involving persons with AD. Steps in this theoretical direction have already been taken by a number of researchers on AD, from Gubrium's early work (1986) and Kitwood's argument that individuals with AD still are persons (Kitwood 1997), to studies of language and interaction in the 1990s (Ramanathan 1997; Hamilton 1994), to the more recent work of Sabat (2001) and others.

Such an approach would also be connected to a number of partially intersecting traditions in psychology, philosophy, and general social science that take persons doing things together as the paradigmatic case for research. Researchers in the sociocultural tradition, beginning with the Russian psychologist Lev Vygotsky, have always argued that the interaction between persons is the base for the child's (and adult's) cognitive, linguistic, and social development (Bruner 1985; Lave and Wenger 1991; Rogoff 1998). A similar position has been taken by researchers engaged in evolutionary research, suggesting that not only humans but also primates develop through social interaction with others (Tomasello et al. 2005; Enfield and Levinson 2006). In addition, the theoretical foundation of research on the micro-organization of interaction and language use has been the interaction between persons as well as between persons and artifacts (Clark 1996; Goffman 1967; Goodwin 1981; Hutchins 1996). Finally, a number of philosophers have pursued the ideas of shared intentions and joint action as an alternative to more classical individualistic notion of actions (Bratman 1992; Gilbert 1992; Toumela 2007).

Common to all these research traditions is that they start from examples of joint activities, often various kinds of conversations or activities involving talk. This implies a focus on the joint activity, its organization and performance, rather than on the individual and his or her behavior. From a collaborative perspective, the individual and his or her behavior and acts are seen as part of the joint activity. As a consequence, in these traditions the individual is primarily seen as emerging from joint activities and not as an entity that exists either before or outside joint activities.

A theoretical perspective that takes joint action and collaboration as the starting point could most certainly be beneficial for studies of persons with AD in interaction with other persons, particularly how they jointly deal with the consequences of cognitive and linguistic loss. This means that it is not the individual with AD who is the prime focus of studies but rather the activities involving persons in the everyday network and the way these persons jointly take on the problems caused by the progressing disease.

AD is a progressive brain disorder with immediate and specific consequences for collaboration, similar to those of other kinds of brain disorders (Goodwin 2003; Perkins 2007; Mates, Mikesell, and Smith 2010). As such it presents a number of challenges for the participants in joint activities—as well as for theories about joint activities. From a collaborative perspective the changes in a person's brain are of interest when they are noted, defined, and handled in the interaction. This is not an argument for side-stepping what is happening in the brain, but rather an argument for treating the brain as a *social organ*: the brain is central for the multimodal coordination of the collaboration and changes in the brain have consequences in the interaction (cf. Hydén 2013). A further implication is that the individual's loss of abilities is defined and dealt with in the activity and hence is a joint problem, rather than an individual problem.

Joint Activities

Many researchers have used the concept of activity. Levinson's definition captures many of the central theoretical features. He suggests that activities are "goal-defined, socially constituted, bounded events with constraints on participants, setting, and so on, but above all on the kinds of allowable contributions" (Levinson 1992, 69).

What Levinson argues is that activities can basically be seen as events with boundaries that put constraints on participants and actions. Joint activities can be of many different kinds. In some cases people have conversations or cook together and in other cases they are involved in joint problem solving, in connection with, for instance, building a house. Some of these joint activities would be impossible to accomplish without collaboration with other people. Conversation is a good example of an activity that actually requires more than one person for its accomplishment. Other activities could be pursued either by collaboration or by one individual, such as preparing a meal. Some joint activities have more or less clear goals set out beforehand, as in many work-related activities. Others allow some kind of goal to develop, as when deciding what to do in the evening. Still others are more or less an end in themselves, like most dinner conversations. Some joint activities are organized around a coordination of more or less autonomous and complementary contributions, while other activities are organized as collaboration, where the contributions are braided into each other.

Furthermore, some joint activities are occasional and may not be repeated, whereas other activities are part of ongoing, long-term relations and are hence repeated with the same participants many times. As such, some joint activities are actually part of the participants' joint life project or "couplehood" (Hellström, Nolan, and Lundh 2005). Joint activities that are part of life projects of course become especially vulnerable when one of the participants loses his or her ability to actually take part in and accomplish these activities.

In joint activities participants must *coordinate* their actions in a special way. Following Gilbert (1992) and Bratman (1992) it could be argued that the participants share a commitment to the joint activity, in the sense that they constitute what Gilbert calls a "plural subject"; that is, they constitute a "we" that is doing something together. The use of the collective pronoun "we" is often central to the phrases most people would use if queried about what they are doing, either in the middle of the activity or in retrospect, when they account for their actions.

This means that the participants in joint activities constitute themselves as something more than just a collection of individuals who happen to have similar intentions. They are rather persons who in various ways have negotiated what they plan to do, are doing, or have done. In that sense they *share* intentions (Bratman 1993). In some cases the shared intentions come close to more or less clearly stated goals—especially in joint activities that are part of formal organizations. In other cases the shared intentions are more or less equal to the activity as such, as in just spending time together waiting for something else. That is, the goal is to cooperate in order to pass time.

Actions as Contributions

Joint activities advance through individual *actions* that function as *contributions* to the activity. Each contribution has to be noted and understood by the other participant; otherwise, some kind of repair becomes necessary until both participants can accept the (negotiated) meaning of the contribution. One way to facilitate this process is to design contributions in such a way that they fit into the previous contributions while adding something new; that is, contributions generally have to be responsive to what already has occurred but note something new in order not to be a repetition. At the same time, contributions also have to be forward-oriented both in relation to the joint activity and in opening up possibilities for other, new contributions by other participants. In this way the process of making a contribution and negotiating its meaning forms a small *joint action* project with a starting point (the individual action), the negotiation phase (including repair if necessary), and finally the acceptance.

Clark's model could be useful for a closer look at how these joint action projects are organized (Clark 1996). Clark argues that in order for people to do something together, they need to cooperate and coordinate their actions at several levels. First they need to share their *attention*; that is, they need to focus on the same thing, in this case an action (utterance). This joint attention allows the participants to focus on hearing and perceiving *what is said* (or done in other ways). Joint attention and hearing in their turn allow for an *understanding* of the action and eventually the *uptake* of the action, for instance answering a question:

(1) Execution of signal for action ⇒ Establishing and maintaining joint attention
(2) Presentation of action ⇒ Identification of what is said or done
(3) Meaning of action ⇒ Understanding of the action
(4) Projection of action ⇒ Uptake of action or response

Central to this hierarchical action model is that it functions as what Clark calls an *action ladder* (1996, 147 ff). A presupposition of uptake and response to a projected action (4), is that the listener understood the meaning of the projected action (3), which in turn presupposes the hearing of the words spoken or otherwise acted (2), which in turn presupposes that the listener's attention is geared toward and coordinated with the speaker's (1).

It seems that persons with AD may have problems in the interaction at all the steps on Clark's ladder, particularly at the "higher" levels. Interestingly, some research indicates that persons with AD—even in very advanced stages—actually take active part in interaction on the level of establishing joint attention and observing turn-taking (Ripich and Terrell 1988; Hydén 2011b; Samuelsson and Hydén 2011). Persons with dementia more often have problems establishing and negotiating meaning. As a consequence of this the person without AD may have to repeat and reformulate his or her own utterances, or request that the person with AD repeat his or her utterance. This may happen when the person with AD is attentive but has problems hearing what is said due to background noise, or the speaker may have problems articulating (level 2 of Clark's ladder). Often the person without AD may have to suggest interpretations, hypotheses, or possible solutions as a way of constructing shared meaning of contributions, when the person with AD may have heard what is said but not understood the utterance and the speaker may have uttered something with a potentially unclear or difficult meaning.

Mutual Commitment

Sharing intentions in activities also implies sharing a commitment to cooperation. That is, the participants are committed to act in such a way that the intentions or goals of the activity can be achieved. This *procedural commitment* is expressed in the way joint activities progress and implies that the participants must be *mutually supportive*. That is, that they must help each other when they encounter problems in the interaction (Bratman 1992; Clark 1996). Working toward shared ends means that the participants not only must be cooperative in making contributions but also in fulfilling these contributions, which implies that they must help each other to create a shared meaning or understanding of their contributions. This may for instance entail talking in a loud voice if the other person has problems hearing; repeating contributions that were not heard or understood; and repairing, expanding, or explaining other contributions.

There are several potential risks and problems connected with mutual support (Bratman 1992). Some of those are of particular relevance in understanding interactions involving persons with AD. First, there is risk that giving support may jeopardize the supporter's ability to make his or her own contributions. A second risk may be that the person giving support may think that the support costs too much in terms of effort, hence making the joint activity not worth the time or energy. A third problem is that the supportive activity may develop into an almost new activity of its own and hence risk replacing or taking over the original activity—something that might be a problem in certain circumstances. The same kind of problems and risks can be identified for the person needing support: the occasional, repeated, or constant need of support may make the participation in a joint activity such an effort that it is not worth it, thus adding to the risk of not being able to pursue the joint commitment. These risks are evaluated at least in two ways. One is a simple calculation of support efforts against the gains from these efforts, where it may become problematic if the costs are higher than the gains. But there is also an evaluation that is more complicated. The risks may be evaluated in terms of the consequences for the long-term interaction and relationship. That is, giving up supporting interaction may minimize the chances for future interactions and hence redefine the relationship.

AD, Joint Activities, and Scaffolding

Several researchers suggest that persons with AD remain active participants and make compensatory shifts in the conversation in order to facilitate participation in it (Ripich et al. 1991; Gallagher-Thompson et al. 2001). It is important to notice that then the person with AD may only be able to participate using a very diminished and restricted set of communicative resources, including, especially at later stages of the disease, mainly basic bodily actions like gaze or touch. Nevertheless, they are still displaying a "cooperative attitude."

Living with a person with AD or being a caregiver in most cases implies that over time a set of specific problems that emerge in collaboration will become well known and identified by both participants because they are both frequent and recur incessantly. Over time, these problems most likely even increase in frequency and severity as a result of the progressing disease. This means that some of these problems tend to occur irrespective of what the participants do, whereas other problems only occur under certain conditions and in that sense are *potential* problems. As a consequence of the increased number of problems, the need for support in joint activity increases and the participants organize their collaboration so that they are still able to do things jointly. The emergence of this kind of collaborative problem and the way the participants deal with it is central to all studies of joint activities involving persons with AD. This means that it is important to try to describe and understand these problems and supportive adaptations in terms of how the joint activities become organized.

If AD and its consequences are seen from the perspective of joint activities, then a focus must be on how the participants deal with the problems that result from the impairments caused by AD. That is, the idea would be that the disease as such does not automatically result in certain consequences or problems. Rather, the interesting point is what kind of problems people themselves identify in collaborations involving people diagnosed with AD, and what strategies they use to deal with these problems. This would also change the description of the impairment from an individual property to a property of the interacting participants, and from impairment with given consequences to a practical problem in the form of interactional troubles identified by the participants. A review of the research on conversations involving persons with AD indicates a number of problems that are frequently identified (Bohling 1991; Hamilton 1994; Perkins, Whitworth, and Lesser 1998; Ramanathan 1997; Watson, Chenery, and Carter 1999): from problems with *participating* in the interaction and *managing* discourse topics, to problems with *understanding* and making *responses*.

The fact that interactional problems occur frequently and increase in joint activities involving persons with AD makes it necessary to include this aspect in a theoretical framework. As already indicated above, activity theory has mainly dealt with interactional asymmetries that can be conceptualized in terms of novice/expert learning. Although the learning aspect is not obvious in activities including persons with AD, some of the notions suggested in a developmental context still can be of interest. In more general terms, one basic way to deal with actual and potential interactional problems might be to change the division of interactional labor between the participants: the person without AD could make contributions that make it easier for the person with AD to understand and respond to contributions, as well as to make further contributions; the person without AD must then also engage in fairly advanced, extensive, and comprehensive interactional work together with the person with AD in order to establish joint meaning.

This redistribution of activities and responsibilities in interaction in many ways resembles what the developmental psychologist Jerome Bruner called *scaffolding*. Bruner and his colleagues (Wood, Bruner, and Ross 1976) argued that when an adult helps a small child solve a problem (tying shoelaces or solving an arithmetic problem) the adult acts as an "expert" who knows how to accomplish the task, while the child does not. The "expert" constructs a scaffold by arranging tasks, support, and feedback in such a way that the child is able to solve the problem on its own:

> "Scaffolding" is a process that enables the child or novice to solve a problem, carry out a task or achieve a goal which would be beyond his unassisted efforts. This scaffolding consists essentially of the adult "controlling" those elements of the task that are initially beyond the learner's capacity, thus permitting him to concentrate upon and complete only those elements that are within his range of competence. (90)

There are at least three problems with the original model suggested by Bruner et al. in relation to activities involving persons with AD. First, the model exclusively focused on situations with a limited number of possible solutions (the toys used in the experimental situation had to be built in certain ways). In interactional situations where people are making conversation, telling stories, or cooking together, the possible options are in many cases more open.

Second, their formulation was also based on a situation constructed in such a way that the roles were fixed (tutor and pupil) by the fact that the tutor was the "holder" of the solution. This could be interpreted to mean that the learner had a more passive role, as the "receptor" of instructions (cf. the criticism of Rogoff 1998). A similar everyday situation would be when one person tries to help another person remember a specific event by suggesting cues. In that situation the helper might be conceived of as the expert knower, while in actuality the participants have to find a solution among themselves in order to be able to proceed with what they are doing. This means that we will have a situation where both participants have to be very active in trying to find and negotiate the meaning of the contribution. In other words, in most everyday situations roles are more open and flexible than in the experiment devised by Bruner and his colleagues.

A third critical point has to do with the fact that in the Bruner experiments, "scaffolding" referred to a learning situation: the child had to learn how to solve a specific problem. That is, the activity and the aim or goal of the activity was to learn some new abilities. In conversations involving persons with AD, the problems the participants have to solve are subparts in an ongoing activity with a different aim or goal from that of problem solving. That is, the problem solving is not the goal of the joint activity, but is rather a subactivity organized around the necessary mutual support.

These critical points suggest that all participants have to be regarded as active in attempting to construct a joint meaning in order to pursue their ongoing activity. It also suggests that interactional support should be conceived of not so much in terms of one person supporting another (as discussed above), but rather as of *mutual support*: participants working together in order to achieve a shared understanding of contributions.

Given these reservations and remarks, it is still possible to use Bruner et al.'s metaphor and idea of scaffolding, because meaning-making in conversations, like the problems presented in the experimental situation, could be thought of in terms of problem solving. The participants must work out a shared understanding of each contribution made by the participants in order to proceed with their activity. Scaffolding is based on a renegotiation of the division of interactional work, implying that although both participants are active, the person without AD has the responsibility for setting up tasks and situations, and using semiotic resources, in such a way that it becomes possible for the other person to take part in meaning making.

Types of Scaffolding

By keeping to both Bruner et al.'s original model and to the concept of joint activity, at least two types of scaffolding in collaboration involving persons with AD can be suggested.

(1) Scaffolding that supports participation in joint activity and the selection of *activity frames* (environment and general preconditions for the activity and

format, perspective, wording, topic) that increase chances for participation of the person with dementia.
(2) Scaffolding that increases likelihood for establishing joint meaning and especially scaffolding involving *repair of contributions* that help to produce an acceptance by either of the participants.

One of the most important kinds of scaffolding has to do with the conversational partner's help in *framing, reframing,* and *reminding* about the joint activity. One way to deal with some of the collaborative problems is for the person without AD to be *proactive* by organizing the interaction beforehand in such a way that the risk for certain problems to emerge is minimized. This means thinking ahead: first, being at least one step ahead of the next turns in the interaction; second, imagining and predicting what will happen if nothing is done; third, predicting the possible problems that may emerge; and fourth, finding alternatives, such as changing aspects of the situation, as well as projecting (possible) alternative turns.

Being proactive in this way may involve things like changing certain aspects of the physical and social situation. This could for instance be done by reducing distraction from other stimuli in the environment in order to enlist the attention of the person with AD and help him or her to keep it focused on the joint activity. It could also mean adapting the general pace of the talk, allowing more time for the turn taking as well as other measures that increase the probability for successful participation (Müller and Guendouzi 2005).

Being proactive also implies projecting next turns that are possible for the person with AD to use and hence to continue to participate in the activity. Many persons with AD, especially in the later stages of AD, provide only minimal responses or turns (Hamilton 1994). One way to deal with this situation could be for the person without AD to talk more and in that way minimize the need for contributions by the person with AD. Another, more proactive way, would be to project a possible format of the next turn, for instance, by asking an open-ended question that would give the next speaker the opportunity to answer by telling a story, something that could be difficult for some persons with AD. The opposite would be to use a closed question that just allows for a simple yes or no or some other specific information, often easier for a person with more advanced AD (Mikesell 2009).

Like most other researchers, Mentis et al. found in their study that persons with AD "produced significantly more problematic topic introductions, including tangential shifts and non coherent topic changes" than persons without AD (Mentis, Briggs-Whittaker, and Gramigna 1995, 1061). They also found that persons with AD in general had difficulty in "maintaining topic sequences," often repeating themselves. In other words, persons with AD often have problems with keeping to the ongoing joint activity, for example by suddenly introducing new conversational topics. One way to scaffold the ongoing joint activity can be for the conversational partner to use questions. Perkins, Whitworth, and Lesser (1998) found that listeners tend to use repetitive questions in conversations with people with dementias. Repeating the same question is a way to maintain topical coherence in the conversation and maintain a conversation flow. By using repeated questions around the same topic, it becomes possible both to the elicit responses into the conversation and to stick to the same conversational topic.

A second type of scaffolding has to do with the possibility of negotiating the meaning of new contributions; of special interest here is *repair* of contributions. The emergence of problems in the course of the conversation and attempts to repair these are ubiquitous in all conversations and interactions. The common way to describe the identification and treatment of interactional problems is in terms of repair. According to this view, repairs are summoned in response to some kind of identified trouble or problem in a contribution (utterance) produced by one of the tellers. Either the teller (self) or the listener (other) may indicate that something is problematic. This is generally done through the use of some verbal or nonverbal flag (behavior indicating trouble) either by self or other. Signaling trouble indicates not only trouble but also what is called the trouble source or source of the problem. This may for instance be mentioning an incorrect fact, uttering an unrecognizable sound, producing the wrong word, or underspecifying something. Generally, the current speaker attempts to repair the trouble (self-repair); in some cases, the other may repair by submitting information or supplying a word (other-repair) (Schegloff, Jefferson, and Sacks 1977).

Although the concept of repair is valuable for understanding many cases of repair in ordinary conversations, it has been suggested that this concept becomes problematic in relation to speakers with communicative disabilities (Milroy and Perkins 1992). There are at least three aspects of the dealings with interactional problems in conversations involving persons with AD that challenge the traditional notion of repair in interaction.

First, in conversations between persons without communicative disabilities there is a general preference for persons making problematic utterances to repair those himself or herself (Schegloff, Jefferson, and Sacks 1977). In conversations involving persons with AD, it turns out that much of the repair work connected to their utterances is accomplished by the person without AD, although the problem or trouble indication may be initiated both by self and other (cf. Watson, Chenery, and Carter 1999). This indicates that the person without AD has a fairly important role in the interaction; the functional relation is asymmetric.

Second, repairs become more complex when the repair attempts presented by either participant themselves include a need for repair (cf. Orange, Lubinski, and Higginbotham 1996). Several sequences may have to be added on to the original sequence.

Third, repair that involves persons with communicative disabilities like AD are often elaborate and involve many turns (Orange Lubinski, and Higginbotham 1996). In many cases attempts to self-repair by the person with AD may require a quite extended number of turns involving the need for repair support by the other person. Here it is less meaningful to use the distinction between self- and other-repair, because the repair is a consequence of extended and elaborate interaction.

It may be more meaningful to reconceptualize the idea of repair in interaction involving persons with AD as *extended, collaborative repair episodes involving scaffolding*. Extended, collaborative repairs are fairly extended subactivities of the joint activity, involving more than three interactional turns. Extended, collaborative repairs take up much of the participant's time and effort and also form a fairly delimited part of the activity with a beginning and end, and thus constitute an *episode* of the activity. Extended, collaborative repair episodes are less dependent on the distinctions between self and other, initiator and repairer, but are better seen as a joint, *collaborative work* of the participants striving for mutual understanding of contributions and hence to complete the activity.

Finally, central to extended, collaborative repair is its character of *joint problem solving*. Participants are facing a problem concerning meaning which they have to solve in order to be able to pursue their joint activity. This also implies that the extended, collaborative repair work involves the participants' creative abilities: they have to set up the problem (the joint understanding) in such a way that makes it solvable for them, allowing them to find solutions by using various semiotic resources (words, nonverbal vocalization, gestures, and so forth).

Oswald and Linda Revisited

This chapter ends with a return to the beginning and hence to Oswald and Linda—an example of *possibilities*: what a person with dementia actually can do together with other persons, rather than what they cannot do. Oswald, like most persons with AD, lives with another person. Living together implies doing things together: discussing, passing time with small talk, cooking together, remembering both the recent past as well as the distant past. The example starting this chapter showed Oswald and Linda involved in a joint activity: telling the story about the life together. Framing their storytelling theoretically as a joint activity implies that the cognitive and linguistic losses connected with AD, and the coping with these, is something that involve all persons in the network—both

Oswald and Linda, not just Oswald (Chambers 2009). Doing things together presupposes that people support and help each other in order to accomplish what they are doing. The example also suggests that the support often has the character of a scaffolded interaction—and that scaffolding can be of many kinds ranging from support of joint activity to support of joint actions. By scaffolding the collaboration both participants may successfully be able to jointly tell a story about the shared past.

Acknowledgments

The research presented in this chapter has been supported by a generous research grant from the Swedish *Riksbankens Jubileumsfond* (M10-0187:1).

References

Blonder, Lee X., Eva D. Kort, and Frederick A. Schmitt. 1994. "Conversational Discourse in Patients with Alzheimer's Disease." *Journal of Linguistic Anthropology* 4: 50–71.
Bohling, Hollis R. 1991. "Communication with Alzheimer's Patients: An Analysis of Caregiver Listening Patterns." *International Journal of Aging and Human Development* 33: 249–267.
Bratman, Michael E. 1992. "Shared Cooperative Activity." *The Philosophical Review* 101: 327–341.
Bratman, Michael E. 1993. "Shared Intention." *Ethics* 104: 97–113.
Bruner, Jerome. 1985. *Child's Talk. Learning to Use Language.* New York: W.W. Norton & Co.
Clark, Herbert H. 1996. *Using Language.* New York: Cambridge University Press.
Chambers, Todd. 2009. "Toward a Naturalized Narrative Bioethics." In *Naturalized Bioethics. Toward Responsible Knowing and Practice*, edited by H. Lindemann, M. Verkerk, and M. U. Walker. New York: Cambridge University Press.
Enfield, Nigel J., and Stephan C. Levinson, editors. 2006. *Roots of Human Sociality. Culture, Cognition and Interaction.* Oxford: Berg.
Gallagher-Thompson, Dolores, Pamela G. Dal Canto, Theodore Jacob, and Larry W. Thompson. 2001. "A Comparison of Marital Interaction Patterns between Couples in Which the Husband Does or Does Not Have Alzheimer's Disease." *Journals of Gerontology: Social Sciences* 56B: S140–S150.
Gilbert, Margaret. 1992. *On Social Facts.* London: Routledge.
Goffman, Erving. 1967. *Interaction Ritual. Essays on Face-to-Face Behavior.* New York: Doubleday.
Goodwin, Charles. 1981. *Conversational Organization: Interaction between Speakers and Hearers.* New York: Academic Press.
Goodwin, Charles. 2003. "Conversational Frameworks for the Accomplishment of Meaning in Aphasia." In *Conversation and Brain Damage*, edited by Charles Goodwin, 90–116. Oxford: Oxford University Press.
Gubrium, Jaber F. 1986. *Oldtimers and Alzheimer's: The Descriptive Organization of Senility.* Greenwich, CT: JAI Press.
Hamilton, Heidi E. 1994. *Conversations with an Alzheimer's Patient. An Interactional Sociolinguistic Study.* New York: Cambridge University Press.
Hellström, Ingrid, Michael Nolan, and Ulla Lundh. 2005. "We Do Things Together: A Case Study of Couplehood in Dementia." *Dementia* 4: 7–22.
Hutchins, Edwin. 1996. *Cognition in the Wild.* Cambridge: MIT Press.

Hydén, Lars-Christer. 2011a. "Narrative Collaboration and Scaffolding in Dementia." *Journal of Aging Studies* 25: 339–347.
Hydén, Lars-Christer. 2011b. "Non-verbal Vocalizations, Dementia and Social Interaction." *Communication and Medicine* 8: 135–144.
Hydén, Lars-Christer. 2013. "Towards an Embodied Theory of Narrative and Storytelling." In *The Travelling Concept of Narrative*, edited by M. Hyvärinen, M. Hatavara, and L. C. Hydén. Amsterdam/Boston: John Benjamins.
Kemper, Susan, Kelly Lyons, and Cheryl Anagnopoulos. 1995. "Joint Storytelling by Patients with Alzheimer's Disease and Their Spouses." *Discourse Processes* 20: 205–217.
Kitwood, Tom. 1997. *Dementia Reconsidered: The Person Comes First*. Philadelphia: Open University Press.
Lave, Jean, and Etienne Wenger. 1991. *Situated Learning. Legitimate Peripheral Participation*. New York: Cambridge University Press.
Levinson, Stephan C. 1992. "Activity Types and Language." In *Talk at Work. Interaction in Institutional Settings*, edited by Paul Drew and John Heritage, 66–100. Cambridge: Cambridge University Press.
Mates, Andrea W., Lisa Mikesell, and Michael Sean Smith. 2010. *Language, Interaction, and Frontotemporal Dementia: Reverse Engineering the Social Mind*. London: Equinox.
Mentis, Michelle, Jan Briggs-Whittaker, and Gary D. Gramigna. 1995. "Discourse Topic Management in Senile Dementia of the Alzheimer's Type." *Journal of Speech and Hearing Research* 38: 1054–1066.
Mikesell, Lisa. 2009. "Conversational Practices of a Frontotemporal Dementia Patient and His Interlocutors." *Research on Language and Social Interaction* 42: 135–162.
Milroy, Lesley, and Lisa Perkins. 1992. "Repair Strategies in Aphasic Dialogue: Towards a Collaborative Model." *Clinical Linguistics and Phonetics* 6: 27–40.
Müller, Nicole, and Jaqueline A. Guendouzi. 2005. "Order and Disorder in Conversation: Encounters with Dementia of the Alzheimer's Type." *Clinical Linguistics and Phonetics* 19: 393–404.
Orange, John B., Rosmary B. Lubinski, and D. Jeffery Higginbotham. 1996. "Conversational Repair by Individuals With Dementia of the Alzheimer's Type." *Journal of Speech and Hearing Research* 39: 881–895.
Perkins, Lisa, Anne Whitworth, and Ruth Lesser. 1998. "Conversing in Dementia: A Conversation Analytic Approach." *Journal of Neurolinguistics* 11: 33–53.
Perkins, Michael. 2007. *Pragmatic Impairment*. Cambridge: Cambridge University Press.
Ramanathan, Vai. 1997. *Alzheimer Discourse. Some Sociolinguistic Dimensions*. Mahwah, NJ: Lawrence Erlbaum Associates.
Ripich, Danielle, and Brenda Terrell. 1988. "Patterns of Discourse Cohesion and Coherence in Alzheimer's Disease." *Journal of Speech and Hearing Disorders* 53: 8–15.
Ripich, Danielle, Diane Vertes, Peter Whitehouse, Sarah Fulton, and Barbara Ekelman. 1991. "Turn-taking and Speech Act Patterns in the Discourse of Senile Dementia of the Alzheimer's Type Patients." *Brain and Language* 40: 330–343.
Rogoff, Barbara. 1998. "Cognition as a Collaborative Process." In *Handbook of Child Psychology, Vol. 2: Cognition, Perception, and Language*, edited by D. Kuhn and R. S. Siegler, 679–744. New York: Wiley.
Sabat, Steve R. 2001. *Experience of Alzheimer's Disease. Life Through a Tangled Veil*. Oxford: Blackwell.
Samuelsson, Christina, and Lars-Christer Hydén. 2011. "Intonational Patterns of Non-verbal Vocalizations in People with Dementia." *American Journal of Alzheimer's Disease and Other Dementias* 26: 563–572.
Schegloff, Emanuel A., Gail Jefferson, and Harvey Sacks. 1977. "The Preference for Self-Correction in the Organization of Repair in Conversation." *Language* 53: 361–382.
Tomasello, Michael, Malinda Carpenter, Josep Call, Tanya Behne, and Henrike Moll. 2005. "Understanding and Sharing Intentions: The Origins of Cultural Cognition." *Behavioral and Brain Sciences* 28: 675–735.

Toumela, R. 2007. *The Philosophy of Sociality: The Shared Point of View*. New York: Oxford University Press.

Usita, Paula M., Ira E. Hyman, and Keith C. Herman. 1998. "Narrative Intentions: Listening to Life Stories in Alzheimers Disease." *Journal of Aging Studies* 12: 185–198.

Watson, Caroline M., Helen J. Chenery, and Michelle S. Carter. 1999. "Analysis of Trouble and Repair in the Natural Conversations of People with Dementia of the Alzheimers Type." *Aphasiology* 13: 195–218.

Wood, David, Jerome Bruner, and Gail Ross. 1976. "The Role of Tutoring in Problem Solving." *Journal of Child Psychology and Psychiatry* 17: 89–100.

10

Comprehension in Interaction: Communication at a Day-care Center

CAMILLA LINDHOLM

Introduction

Dementias are a major reason for impairment among the elderly, ultimately causing hospitalization. However, before they enter long-term care, older persons with dementia may live in their own home or with family members and take part in day-care services once or several times a week. Attending these sessions is well suited to elderly people with mild or moderate dementia, who can benefit from the support, activities, and entertainment offered in such a group setting. The purpose of day care is to promote the well-being of the elderly and to provide support to their caregivers.

The day-care center is not a mainstream clinical space but a setting in which the institutional element, while present, is de-emphasized. Many of the activities presented as pastimes, such as playing games and reading the newspaper, are, in fact, therapeutic, aimed at maintaining or rehabilitating the social and interaction skills of the elderly. Thus, the day-care center constitutes a hybrid communication environment in which the health-care personnel strive for a balance between their institutional agenda and a social role of a conversation coparticipant (cf. Sarangi 2008).

Working with a conversation-analysis–inspired research method[1] to examine video-recorded interactions, this chapter explores the communication environment at a Finnish-Swedish day-care center. The study reported upon here concentrated on how elderly persons with dementia express difficulties in comprehension and hearing. By investigating these problems and how they are solved, this chapter creates a picture of the day-care center as a communication arena. The discussion is organized as follows. First, I give an introduction to the day-care center as a communication milieu. Then, the next section examines how people with dementia request clarification and how they respond to the healthy coparticipants' attempts to repair an interaction problem. The chapter concludes with a discussion of comprehension in interaction. Comprehension abilities and disabilities are demonstrated to be as much a collective production as they are consequences of preserved or lost abilities in the person with dementia.

The Day-care Center as a Communication Milieu

Communication challenges of various types can be intensified in institutional encounters between persons with communication difficulties and their caregivers (Wray 2008). First, we have the care recipient with a neurological disease that affects language skills. The care recipient's language production and comprehension both are impaired, which influences such skills as naming objects, introducing a new topic, and comprehending spoken language (starting, for example, with impaired understanding of complex sentences and proceeding to general problems in sentence comprehension) (cf. Bryan and Maxim 2006; Bayles and Tomoeda 2007).

Here, the day-care setting introduces additional challenges. Many persons with dementia suffer from hearing loss or impairment, creating difficulties in an environment with background noise (Bayles and Tomoeda 2007; cf. Caissie and Rockwell 1994). Many of them have attention deficits, which render it difficult to concentrate on several stimuli at the same time (Collette et al. 1999; Baddeley et al. 2001) and frustrate their attempts to make out a message produced simultaneously with another activity (if, for instance, a nurse asks a question while the person with dementia is walking around in the room) or to attend to group conversation (Lindholm 2012). Additionally, groups in the day-care center setting are often heterogeneous, consisting of persons with several types of communication difficulties. Ideally, the groups should be homogenous and be composed of people with equal opportunities to participate in the activities at the center. Regardless of attention to these ideals, it is often difficult to establish entirely homogenous groups, at least if the clients are recruited from a linguistic minority[2] (cf. Lindholm 2012).

Investigating Comprehension Problems at a Day-care Center

Clearly, the day-care center constitutes an environment in which communication challenges, among them comprehension problems, can accumulate. At the same time, however, admitting to linguistic incompetence, such as comprehension difficulties, is a potentially face-threatening activity. This is one important factor in problems of understanding usually remaining beneath the surface in the conversation (cf. Wilkinson 2007), with one result being that the researcher might find it difficult to assess whether the participants really experience the situation as problematic or, in contrast, he or she is making this interpretation merely on account of prior knowledge of the situation as involving people with language deficits (Hamilton 1994). To overcome these methodological difficulties, I have chosen to focus my analysis on situations in which the elderly pose requests for clarification (of the "what," "huh," "who," and "where" type) and thereby show that they have encountered an interaction problem. In this, I follow the research orientation outlined by Hamilton (187): "An examination of the participants' requests for clarification can provide us with important information 'straight from the horse's mouth' regarding problems in the sense-making process as the participants identify them." Requests for clarification are typically preceded in the conversational turn-taking by "trouble turns" and followed by attempts to rectify, or "repair," the initial trouble, a process outlined in the following schematic sequence:

(1) Trouble sequence 1

　　　Trouble turn (speaker A)　　　　　　*He's a teacher*
　　　Request for clarification (speaker B)　*What?*
　　　Repair turn (speaker A)　　　　　　　*He's a teacher*

Here, the clarification request is the open initiator "What?" targeting the whole previous utterance as the trouble source (cf. Drew 1997). The requests for clarification can consist of various kinds of items (Schegloff, Jefferson, and Sacks 1977; Hamilton 1994; Orange, Lubinski, and Higginbotham 1996; Watson, Chenery, and Carter 1999; Schegloff 2000)—for example, of question words and forms (e.g., "what" and "huh") or of partial/full repeating or paraphrasing of the trouble turn. Above, the repair turn consists of (pure) repetition of the trouble turn "He's a teacher." However, pure repetitions are relatively infrequent (Ridell 2008, 137); even when lexically identical to the trouble turn, the repetition usually is uttered at a slower pace and thus differs from the trouble turn. Of course, neither are repair turns always repetitions. In other types of repair turns, speaker A adds new information or reformulates the contents of the trouble turn. Repair turns express how speaker A has interpreted B's request for clarification (Ridell 2008). In sequence 1, we can hypothesize that A has interpreted "What?" as a marker of a hearing problem and therefore repeated the whole trouble turn. In the repair turn, A thus expresses an attempt to solve an interaction problem. How, then, does B show whether he or she has really understood the repair turn? What happens after the repair turn?

(2) Trouble sequence 2

Trouble turn (speaker A)	*He's a teacher*
Request for clarification (speaker B)	*What?*
Repair turn (speaker A)	*He's a teacher*
Turn 4: Reaction to repair turn (speaker B)	*Oh*

Sequence 2 contains a fourth turn, in which speaker B can express improved understanding more or less explicitly. In sequence 2, B reacts to A's repair turn with the news-receipt token "Oh," demonstrating that B was previously unfamiliar with the information provided in the repair turn. Analyzing how elderly persons with dementia demonstrate comprehension in these fourth turns in trouble sequences is fruitful, since fourth turns have the capacity of expressing comprehension and concretizing problems related to the notion of comprehension in interaction. Comprehension problems and their resolution are demonstrated to be as much products of the interaction as they are automatic consequences of lost or preserved abilities in the person with dementia (Guendouzi and Müller 2006, 104, drawing on the ideas of Perkins 2007 and 2008).

Expressing Comprehension Implicitly: The Conversation Moves Forward?

In turn 4, following the repair turn, the elderly person has an opportunity to express whether he or she understood the repair turn. Thus, the fourth turn shows whether the person with dementia was capable of making sense of the repair turn: he or she can demonstrate understanding in a more or less explicit way (Ridell 2008). When turn 4 contains merely an answer to the trouble turn, understanding is expressed implicitly: the conversation simply moves on, without focusing on the comprehension problem. In other cases, the possibility of understanding is demonstrated more explicitly and presented to the conversation partner for confirmation (Ridell 2008, 151). Let us take a look at a third extract (3), in which nurse Gunilla (G) and elderly man Fredrik (F) are sitting on the sofa, talking about Fredrik's siblings and their occupations. In line 1, Gunilla makes a statement about Fredrik's career as a lawyer, which later becomes the topic for an additional question: "was it daddy's wish" (line 5).

(3) Daddy's wish³

01	G:	yes you became a lawyer
02	F:	yes
03	G:	.yeah
04		(1.1)
05	G:	was it daddy's wish
06	F:	(what) ((places his hand behind his ear))
07	G:	was it daddy's wish
08		(0.7)
09	**F:**	**daddy's wish**
10	G:	mm
11	**F:**	**well no I can't say [that**
12	G:	[no
13		**I guess there were (.hh) a few**
14		**discussions [heh heh**
15	G:	[mm (0.6) and well [you must have been a little
16	F:	[yes
17	G:	interested too in the judicial path

Gunilla's question in line 5 fails to receive an answer. Instead, Fredrik reacts by asking "what," simultaneously leaning forward and placing his hand behind his ear. Thereby, he is both verbally and nonverbally signaling a need for clarification (cf. Pajo forthcoming). As mentioned above, open clarification requests such as "what" do not target a specific trouble source. Since Gunilla responds by producing an identical repeat of the trouble turn, we can hypothesize that she has interpreted "what" and the change in Fredrik's posture as indicating a problem with grasping the utterance as a whole.

What exactly happens in Fredrik's turn 4, in line 9? This turn consists of repetition of the phrase "daddy's wish," from Gunilla's previous turns. Whether partial repeating of this type actually demonstrates comprehension explicitly (as argued by Ridell 2008, 151) is disputable. On one hand, Fredrik's repeat presents a hypothesis about, and at least partial understanding of, the contents of the previous utterance. At the same time, however, he addresses the repeat to Gunilla for confirmation. Fredrik is simultaneously demonstrating understanding and seeking verification of his understanding. Gunilla confirms his hypothesis with "mm" (line 10), after which Fredrik gives an answer to the question of whether his father had wanted him to be a lawyer. This elaboration, starting in line 11, demonstrates in-depth comprehension: Fredrik is capable of providing a response to the original question, and the conversation moves forward, with Gunilla (in lines 15–17) making another comment on

Fredrik's occupation, in which she rephrases the assumption she expressed in the trouble turn.

Coparticipants usually treat expanded turn 4 reactions, such as the one in line 11, as signaling the successful solving of a problem in the interaction. This is not always the case: expanded turn 4 reactions are sometimes still treated as insufficient indicators of comprehension. In these cases, the notion of comprehension in interaction turns out to be problematic, as illustrated in the following extracts (4–6). These extracts have in common that the elderly person with dementia in his turn 4 reactions simultaneously expresses both comprehension and engagement in another activity than that of the previous speaker. As a result of this, the previous speaker then comments on the turn 4 reactions in ways showing that these reactions are deemed insufficient responses. In the extract below, the participants are having lunch when Gunilla (G) makes a statement about the gravy, looking at her plate. Her utterance does not address anyone in particular, yet her nurse colleague Riikka (R) acts as the primary recipient by posing a question on the current topic (in line 3). Before Gunilla responds to Riikka, however, Didrik (D) enters the conversation.

(4) The gravy

```
01   G:   it's special this gravy
02        (1.2)
03   R:   is it good
04        (2.7)
05   D:   the gravy ((turns towards Gunilla))
06   G:   the gravy (1.9, Gunilla looks at Didrik's plate) tastes
          special (.)
07        but it's [good
08   D:   [yes there are are (1.2) two drops at least
09   G:   (hh) mm:
10        (0.6)
11   G:   she did put a lot it has sunk into the rice (.) I did see that
          [Riikka
12   D:   [oh
13   G:   pu[t a lot [of gravy
14   R:       [mm:
15   D:            [*oh yes*
```

In line 5, Didrik partially repeats Gunilla's previous turn, with his "the gravy" placing stress on the first syllable and thus signaling that he treats this referent as something problematic (Selting 1996: *astonished questions*). He also leans forward

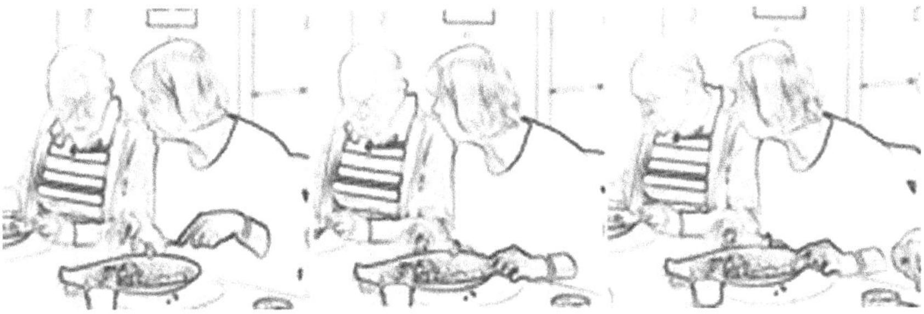

Figure 10.1 Gunilla and Didrik looking at the soup

toward Gunilla (Figure 10.1A). Gunilla responds to him both verbally and nonverbally; she repeats "the gravy" and turns toward Didrik's plate (Figure 10.1B). By changing her physical posture and the direction of her gaze, Gunilla encourages Didrik to direct his attention to his food, and he indeed does so (Figure 10.1C). Once she has drawn his attention to the plate, she provides additional information about the gravy. Gunilla performs three actions in her turn in lines 6–7: (1) she helps Didrik to localize the referent he asked about, (2) she repeats the content of line 1 ("the gravy tastes special"), and (3) she adds another element ("but it's good")—which is a response to Riikka's question in line 3. In her repair turn, Gunilla manages to involve both coparticipants in the conversation.

Didrik's response in line 8 demonstrates at least partial comprehension, since he manages to show recognition of the referent "gravy." Yet in his response he fails to perform the preferred activity. The gravy Gunilla was talking about is a referent all participants are supposed to have mutual access to, since they are eating the same food. She made an assessment of this food, and the preferred subsequent action is a second assessment (Pomerantz 1984). However, Didrik does not provide an assessment. Instead he looks at his plate, saying that there is only a small amount of gravy on his plate. This apparently is to account for his inability to make a comment on the gravy. Gunilla responds by saying that the gravy Riikka gave him has been absorbed by the food. This is an intriguing case, since the nurses very rarely correct the elderly participants' understanding, even in cases of confabulation (Lindholm 2011). Why is it, then, so important for Gunilla to challenge Didrik's understanding? Gunilla seems to be treating Didrik's contribution as a potential complaint that needs to be challenged; apparently, he can identify only a minimal amount of gravy on his plate. Since the nurses are representatives of the institution and in this case Riikka has more direct responsibility for providing the care recipients with food, Didrik's perception can probably be interpreted as calling into question the nurses' professional actions, so Gunilla needs to refute the possible complaint in order to express professional loyalty (Heinemann 2009).

In the next extract, the participants are engaged in a game of proverbs. These games are used at the day-care center as a memory- and language-stimulating activity (for a more detailed discussion of this activity, Lindholm and Wray 2012). The game material consists of a pack of cards with fixed Swedish-language sayings. In the game, a nurse reads the first part of a proverb aloud, creating a slot that the care recipients are intended to fill in by producing the second part. The nurse reads the relevant card to verify whether the response provided is correct. Sometimes the nurse also refers to the text on the cards as an external source of authority, stating the correct answer. If no one is able to produce the item searched for, the nurses usually start giving hints about the correct response. In extract 5, the participants have engaged in lengthy discussion about the saying "in the shallowest waters, the biggest fish swim," and Didrik (D) and Martin (M) have collaborated to produce the sought-for answer. In line 1, the nurse, Ingrid (I), repeats this saying.

(5)   The biggest fish

```
01   I:   in the shallowest waters, the biggest fish swim
02   M:   #yes#
03        (0.3)
04   D:   yes
05        (0.3)
06   I:   what does that mean
07        (0.3)
08   M:   the biggest fish
09        (0.3)
10   I:   yes
11        (0.4)
12   M:   that's the biggest (.h) well biggest
13        is always the best
14        (0.4)
15   D:   (.h).yes
16   I:   but what does it refer to in the shallowest
17        waters what
```

In line 6, Ingrid asks Didrik and Martin "what does that mean." Martin responds (in line 8) by requesting clarification. He repeats the string "the biggest fish," working from a hypothesis about the element in need of clarification and checking what the pronoun "that" referred to. Previous studies (Almor et al. 1999; Orange and Colton-Hudson 1998; Hopper 2001; Bayles 2003; Bayles and Tomoeda 2007) have demonstrated that interpreting pronouns and understanding what these refer to often create difficulties for persons with dementia. This is the case here. Ingrid provides a minimal confirmation (in line 10), after which Martin continues by explaining how he understands "the biggest fish" and, indeed, why big fish are desirable (lines 12–13). The sequence could have come to an end here but an unsatisfying one from the standpoint of the game. Ingrid continues the exchange by posing another question on the topic, now bringing in the description "in the shallowest waters," and, thus, her whole turn in line 1, as the element that needs to be explained. The prolongation of the repair sequence appears to be caused by Ingrid's confirmation of Martin's clarification request in line 8. Through that confirmation, he has interpreted "the biggest fish" as the item that needs to be clarified. Therefore, Martin goes on by explaining the meaning of this word string. The notion of comprehension is somewhat problematic in this extract too—Martin extends the topic in line with the outcome of his request for clarification. In doing so, he displays comprehension of the previous local context but not necessarily of the whole sequence. Extract 5 is an example of a phenomenon Guendouzi and Müller (2006, 109) point out in conversations with elderly people who have dementia: the conversations typically contain sequences with many clarifying questions. This extract also shows how trouble in interaction results from the activities of both participants, not only from the person with dementia.

Sequence 6, below, serves as another example showcasing the complexity of comprehension in interaction. The extract, from the same game as extract 5, starts with a successful contribution by Didrik (D), who encounters problems later in the sequence.

(6)   He hit the head of the nail (equivalent to the English "he hit the nail on the head")

```
01    I:    he hit the head
02          (0.7)
03    M:    o[h
04    D:    [of the [nail
05    M:    [((laughs))
06    I:    *yes*
07          (0.5)
08    I:    well that must have hurt
09          (1.0)
10    I:    ((laugh[s))
11    D:    [yes
12          (4.3)
13    D:    t[he nail then [or [what
```

14	I:	[be- [YES *the nail*
15	M:	[yes
16	**D:**	**I think [this nail doesn't have**
17	M:	[yes
18	**D:**	**that many nerves**
19	I:	((giggles))
20		(1.1)
21	I:	((laugh[s))] *no but maybe the head* (heh)
22	D:	[((laughs))]
23		(0.4)
24	D:	yes
25		(1.0)
26	I:	yes no I don't think *the nail maybe* (0.8)(heh)*got hu[rt*
27	D:	[oh
28		(1.8)
29	I:	better flee than,

The beginning of extract 6 follows the rules of the proverb game: Ingrid (I) produces the incomplete first part of the saying, and Didrik (D) completes the saying, successfully (in line 4). The problems start in line 8, when Ingrid makes a joke, playing with the contents of the saying. This is a fairly advanced joke, with its wordplay referring to an unlikely but possible interpretation of the original Swedish-language utterance "han träffade huvudet på spiken." This utterance can mean both "He hit the head of the nail" and "He hit his head on the nail," with the latter interpretation being both grammatically and semantically odd. When uttering this playful utterance, Ingrid looks directly at Didrik, addressing him as the primary recipient. Ingrid's tone is playful, and also she starts laughing, further signaling that her utterance is to be interpreted as humor (Jefferson 1979). Didrik's next contributions (in lines 11 and 13) signal problems in understanding her joke.

The misunderstandings continue as the conversation moves forward. Didrik's question in line 13 seems to be asking Ingrid to explain her previous utterance; he wants to know whether the nail got hurt. Ingrid, however, provides not an explanation but merely a confirming response (in line 14). Accordingly, Didrik develops the topic of the nail feeling pain (in lines 16 and 18). Here, Didrik demonstrates understanding in the sense that he is capable of continuing with the previous topic and commenting on Ingrid's utterance in line 8. Yet the understanding he expresses is not enough. The comprehension problem here is related to the dichotomy between seriousness and nonseriousness (cf. Schegloff 1987); Didrik failed to notice that Ingrid was joking, and he attempts to explain to her why it is unlikely that the nail got hurt. When Ingrid starts laughing, it seems as if she is treating Didrik's comment as a joke, not that she is pointing to a comprehension problem. Later (in line 21), she provides an explanation, however; the person hitting the nail could have hurt his head. This is a way of adjusting Didrik's conceptions without letting the correction become the explicit business of the interaction (Jefferson 1987: *embedded correction*). The correction is further softened in that Ingrid is smiling and laughing as she produces it. Ingrid's effort to get Didrik back on track turns out to be unsuccessful. He responds with a minimal "yes," not indicating understanding of the playfulness of Ingrid's utterance. Because Didrik fails to show comprehension and appreciation of Ingrid's joke, she, smiling, makes another attempt to point out the unlikeliness of the nail getting hurt. Another minimal response, "oh" (in line 27), follows. At this point, Ingrid stops initiating more explanations. She moves on to the next topic.

This extract illustrates extreme communication difficulties. In line 4, Didrik is capable of successfully completing the saying that Ingrid initiated. His problems are related instead to Ingrid's wordplay in line 8; he does not understand her playful utterance, although he works to achieve understanding (in lines 13 and 16–18). Ingrid makes several attempts to achieve joint understanding (lines 21 and 26), but the sequence still ends with Didrik indicating a lack of comprehension (line 27) and Ingrid continuing to the next saying (line 29).

Extract 6 is an excellent example of a situation wherein the elderly person's success is turned into a failure because of the healthy coconversationalist's overly advanced playing with words. One reason for Didrik's comprehension difficulties may be that persons with dementia usually have problems in comprehending irony, sarcasm, and other indirect ways of speaking (Rapp and Wild 2011). Another reason might be that the game operates in an alternative world with a fixed set of rules. Lindholm and Wray (2012) point out that games will be incomprehensible to anyone who fails to make the transition to the game world—for example, because of having forgotten that a game is being played. Sometimes it is difficult for persons with dementia to make this transition. In extract 6, it is the nurse who, with her wordplay, chooses to break out of the game world. This transition may be confusing for Didrik, who might not be capable of stepping outside the game world to enter a world of wordplay for a short while.

Comprehension in interaction is a complex issue. Sometimes an elderly person provides a response to the trouble turn in which he or she expresses recognition of the topic and of the turn-taking rules in interaction but in which there may be problems in understanding or grasping the topic or activity at a global level (as in extract 5) or in differentiating between a serious and a nonserious mode (as in extract 6). The matter of comprehension appears to be, above all, an issue of performing the activity that is suitable in the context, such as responding to an assessment with a second assessment or to a joke with laughter. This underlines that understanding is best seen as a sequential matter: "[T]he trouble source, lies, rather, in the perceived lack of 'fit' between that turn and its prior sequence" (Drew 1997, 98). Trouble is an emergent phenomenon in interaction, caused by the actions of multiple participants (Guendouzi and Müller 2006). This is also the case when elderly people demonstrate understanding by using news-receipt tokens, which is the topic of the next section.

Expressing Comprehension Explicitly: News-Receipt Tokens

Sometimes people with dementia react to repair turns by producing news-receipt tokens, such as "oh" (see example 2; cf. Heritage 1984; Ridell 2008). Discussing cases of tokens of news receipt yields further hints as to how comprehension is negotiated in interaction. The following extract depicts a situation in which the participants are seated at the lunch table at the day-care center and Gunilla is telling the others about her sister who wants to have her teeth bleached.

(7) Bleaching teeth

```
01    G:    I have a sister who lives in Stockholm [...]
02          now I talked to her on Midsummer and she
03          had now decided that she'll bleach
04          her teeth
05          (1.0)
06    R:    *(hh)*
07          (0.5)
08    I:    *hh*
09          (1.3)
10    D:    ((clears throat)) she'll what ((turns towards Gunilla))
11    G:    she'll *bleach* her teeth
12          (0.3)
13    D:    *oh*
14    (0.7) ((Gunilla shakes her head, looks at Ingrid))
15    R:    *(h)*
16          (0.5)
17    I:    I had a buddy who did who bought just
18          through some TV shop or something
```

When talking about her sister, Gunilla (G) is facing Ingrid (I), gazing at her and apparently treating her as the primary recipient of the utterance. Both Ingrid and the researcher (R), who is seated on the other side of the table and therefore invisible in the picture, start laughing. The healthy coparticipants react to Gunilla's utterance as a laughing matter, whereas Didrik (D) asks "she'll what" and turns towards Gunilla. He both verbally and nonverbally shows his willingness to engage in an information exchange in which he was not addressed as the primary recipient. In Goffman's (1981) terminology, Didrik exchanges the role of a bystander and overhearer for that of a ratified recipient, actively involved in the interaction. As her answer, Gunilla repeats the most important contents of her previous utterance, "she'll bleach her teeth" (line 11), simultaneously turning towards Didrik, to her right (Figure 10.2).

Didrik's reaction to Gunilla's repair turn is brief. He only says "oh," smiles, and returns to his prior activity of eating soup. Gunilla does not pay further attention to Didrik; instead, she focuses nonverbally on Ingrid, smiling and looking at her. Gunilla took the single news-receipt token "oh" to be sufficient expression of comprehension. The pattern illustrated here, wherein speaker A stops talking about the previous topic and does not comment on the news-receipt token, is infrequent. More frequently, speaker A continues talking about the previous topic, as in extract 8.

(8) To the barbershop

         01   G: mt (.h) and Martin has got parturi [(FI for "barbershop"]
         02   after one o'clock
         03   (0.8)
         04   M: what do I have
         05   (0.4)
         06   G: parturi [FI for "barbershop"]
         07   (0.8)

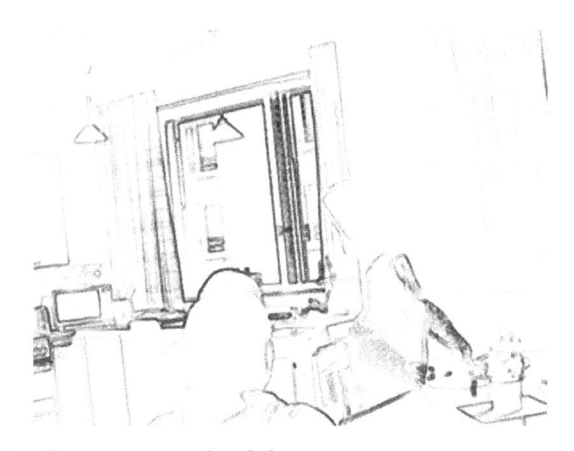

Figure 10.2 Gunilla turning toward Didrik

08	**M:**	**oh**
09	G:	barberare (SW for "barbershop"]
10	M:	no yes
11	G:	yes we'll help you there [one or half past
12	M:	[yes

In extract 8, a single particle expressing a change of state is treated as insufficient indication of understanding. Gunilla (G) is talking about the schedule for the day, and she says that Martin (M) is going to the barber's at one o'clock (lines 1–2). Martin asks for clarification—"what do I have"—and Gunilla responds by repeating the targeted, "barber," element. Martin reacts to the repair turn with a single "oh." Unlike in extract 7, Gunilla does not leave the matter here. She continues by paraphrasing her previous utterance. This paraphrase involves a change of language; she shifts from Finnish to Swedish. The paraphrasing is accompanied by a gesture; Gunilla lifts her hand and makes a circling gesture with her finger near her head, thereby referring to curls while simultaneously looking at Martin, who is sitting opposite her (Figure 10.3). Thus, she uses both verbal and nonverbal means to help Martin understand what she has been talking about.

News-receipt tokens have potential to express comprehension, but usually they are followed by additional utterances in which the nurse continues with the current topic. Many of these continuations question the sufficiency of the comprehension expressed in the token. Unlike Gunilla's clearly corrective paraphrasing in extract 8, it may be impossible to tell whether these follow-up utterances just develop the topic or embody embedded corrections, adding information to ensure the coparticipant's understanding.

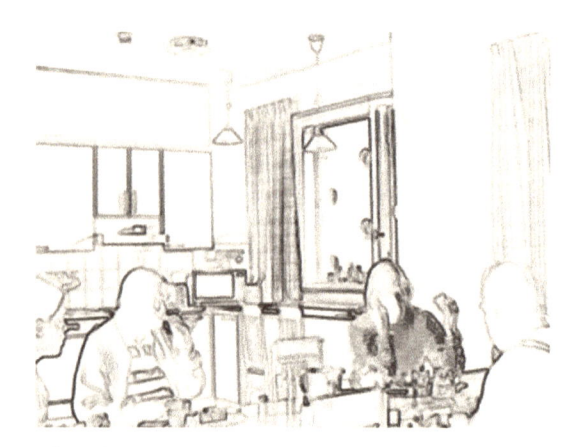

Figure 10.3 Gunilla making circling gesture

Extracts 7 and 8 illustrate a recurring pattern. News-receipt tokens such as "oh" are often treated as sufficient responses when they occur in sequences whose topic is related either to speaker A (as in extract 7, wherein Gunilla was talking about her sister) or to the ongoing situation. Another common feature is that speaker B, who provides the news-receipt token, usually is not the primary addressee of the trouble turn. Instead, speaker A usually is speaking to the whole group and perhaps, above all, to a colleague and the researcher, while the person with dementia, by engaging in the discussion, exchanges the role of a bystander for that of a ratified recipient (as in extract 7). In contrast, those news-receipt tokens treated as insufficient responses are usually produced in sequences in which speaker B is the primary recipient of the trouble turn or when the topic is related to B. We saw this, for example, with extract 8: because the topic is to do with coparticipant B's (i.e., Martin's) schedule, it is important to be sure that he has understood what is going on. This is why Gunilla makes an explicit attempt to ensure Martin understands. The nurses, as the professional caregivers for these elderly people with dementia, decide when the comprehension expressed by the care recipient is sufficient and when the topic is to be addressed further.

Comprehending Comprehension

The day-care center as a communication milieu entails some challenges. One of these difficulties is related to the challenges of multiparty conversation. Sometimes the nurses engage in conversations that are difficult for the dementia-sufferers to follow—for example, because the care recipients have problems in concentrating on several simultaneous stimuli. In these situations, posing requests for clarification may be the dementia-sufferer's only opportunity to contribute to discussion of the topic and to become a ratified participant. We saw examples of this in extracts 4 and 7, with conversation in which an elderly person with dementia engages in discussion in which he was not the primary recipient. In other cases, the elderly people are the primary addressees and need to pose clarification requests if they are to be capable of contributing their thoughts on a topic that concerns them (as in extract 8). Even if the requests for clarification express problems with hearing and comprehension, their use demonstrates the elderly participants' capacity of contributing to the conversations. The requests serve as a resource and often enable the care recipients to follow the topic.

The nurses are more engaged in ensuring the elderly participants' comprehension when the topic is primarily connected to the elderly person. In other cases, when the topic is related to the nurses or to the physical environment, the nurses are more prepared to accept a simple news-receipt token as sufficient response. The nurses appear to have varying expectations in these situations. In cases related to the elderly participants' sphere of life (as in extract 8), the nurses aim at achieving mutual understanding, whereas in other cases (as in extract 7) they are satisfied with maintaining a comfortable atmosphere of small talk (cf. Sidnell 2012). Therefore, minimal contributions by the elderly, or joint attention to a given referent, is regarded as sufficient contribution in the second case.

Day-care service provides stimulation outside the home. Some of the activities involved, however, easily create situations of increasing comprehension problems. In extracts 5 and 6 analyzed above, a person with dementia encountered communication problems due to problems in understanding the ongoing activity, a game with proverbs. The care recipients managed the situation well but encountered problems because of the nurse's failure to pay attention to the clarification requests or to the frame of the game world. In extracts 5 and 6, the trouble arises from the healthy coparticipant's nonadjustment to the person with a deficit, so the trouble can be classified as a property of the interaction itself (cf. Guendouzi and Müller 2006, 115).

The analysis here shows that persons with dementia may retain abilities to request clarification and express comprehension. Comprehension difficulties do not occur as automatic consequences of loss of abilities. Instead, they occur collaboratively in interaction. Elderly persons with dementia are not disabled, isolated individuals but people who are capable of taking turns, engaging in discussion of various topics, and getting involved in communicative and social activities—for example, at the day-care center.

Transcription Symbols

[	Beginning of overlap
]	The point at which overlapping utterances stop overlapping
(0.6)	Interval in the stream of conversation, given in tenths of a second
(.)	Micropause, less than 0.2 seconds
,	Continuing intonation
oh	Emphasis
°oh°	Quiet/muted speech
oh:	Prolongation of a sound
#oh#	Creaky voice
((laughs))	Laughter
(heh)	One laughter particle
oh	"Smiling" voice
(.h)	Inhalation
(h), (hh)	Exhalation
(( ))	Description of the speech or of nonverbal activity

Notes

1. In accordance with the principles of conversation analysis, my analysis is contextual and sequential. Utterances are studied in the context in which they occur, and all conversation details are considered potentially important.
2. Finland is an officially bilingual country with a Swedish-speaking minority that amounts to nearly 300,000 people (5.6% of the country's total population). My data were collected at a day-care center targeting this population.
3. In view of space restrictions, only English-language translations of extracts from the conversations, originally in Swedish, are presented here. All participants in the conversations are assigned Swedish-Finnish pseudonyms, to preserve the feeling of the original data.

References

Almor, Amit, Daniel Kempler, Maryellen C. MacDonald, Elaine S. Andersen, and Lorraine K. Tyler. 1999. "Why Do Alzheimer Patients Have Difficulty with Pronouns? Working Memory, Semantics, and Reference in Comprehension and Production In Alzheimer's Disease." *Brain and Language* 67: 202–227.
Alzheimer's Association. 2012. Accessed January 29, 2013, http://www.alz.org/alzheimers_disease_facts_and_figures.asp.
Baddeley, Alan D., H. A. Baddeley, R. S. Bucks, and G. K. Wilcock. 2001. "Attentional Control in Alzheimer's Disease." *Brain* 124 (8): 1492–1508.
Bayles, Kathryn A. 2003. "Effects of Working Memory Deficits on the Communicative Functioning of Alzheimer's Dementia Patients." *Journal of Communication Disorders* 36: 209–219.
Bayles, Kathryn A., and Cheryl K. Tomoeda. 2007. *Cognitive-Communication Disorders of Dementia*. San Diego: Plural Publishing.
Bryan, Karen, and Jane Maxim, editors. 2006. *Communication Disability in the Dementias*. London: Whurr Publishers.
Caissie, Rachel, and Elaine Rockwell. 1994. "Communication Difficulties Experienced by Nursing Home Residents with a Hearing Loss During Conversation with Staff Members." *JSLPA* 18 (2): 127–134.
Collette, Fabienne, Martial van der Linden, Eric Salmon, and Sophie Bechet. 1999. "Phonological Loop and Central Executive Functioning in Alzheimer's Disease." *Neuropsychologia* 37: 905–918.
Drew, Paul. 1997. "'Open' Class Repair Initiators in Response to Sequential Sources of Trouble in Conversation." *Journal of Pragmatics* 28 (1): 69–101.
Goffman, Erving. 1981. *Forms of Talk*. New York: Pantheon Books.
Guendouzi, Jacqueline, and Nicole Müller. 2006. *Approaches to Discourse in Dementia*. Mahwah, New Jersey: Lawrence Erlbaum.
Hamilton, Heidi E. 1994. "Requests for Clarification As Evidence of Pragmatic Comprehension Difficulty: The Case of Alzheimer's Disease." In *Discourse Analysis and Applications: Studies in Adult Clinical Populations*, edited by Ronald L. Bloom, Loraine K. Obler, Susan DeSanti, and Jonathan S. Ehrlich. Hillsdale, NJ: Lawrence Erlbaum.
Heinemann, Trine. 2009. "Participation and Exclusion in Third Party Complaints." *Journal of Pragmatics* 41 (12): 2435–2451.
Heritage, John. 1984. *Garfinkel and Ethnomethodology*. Cambridge: Polity Press.
Hopper, Tammy. 2001. "Indirect Interventions to Facilitate Communication in Alzheimer's Disease." *Seminars in Speech and Language* 22: 305–315.
Jefferson, Gail. 1979. "A Technique for Inviting Laughter and Its Subsequent Acceptance Declination." In *Everyday Language: Studies in Ethnomethodology*, edited by George Psathas. New York: Irvington Publishers.

Jefferson, Gail. 1987. "On Exposed and Embedded Correction in Conversation." In *Talk and Social Organization*, edited by Graham Button and John R. E. Lee. Clevedon, UK: Multilingual Matters.
Lindholm, Camilla. 2011. "Responsibility and Narrativity in Conversation—the Case of Confabulations." Paper presented at the 12th International Pragmatics Conference, Budapest, July 8, 2011.
Lindholm, Camilla. 2012. "Vuorovaikutuksen haasteita ja mahdollisuuksia—tapaustutkimus muistisairaiden päivätoiminnasta" [Challenges and Opportunities in Interaction—a Case Study from a Day-Care Center for Elderly Persons with Dementia]. In *Haavoittuva keskustelu. Keskustelunanalyyttisia Tutkimuksia Kielellisesti Epäsymmetrisestä Vuorovaikutuksesta*, edited by Leealaura Leskelä and Camilla Lindholm. Helsinki: Kehitysvammaliitto.
Lindholm, Camilla, and Alison Wray. 2012. "Proverbs and Formulaic Sequences in the Language of Elderly People with Dementia." *Dementia* 10 (4): 603–623.
Orange, Joseph B., and Angela Colton-Hudson. 1998. "Enhancing Communication in Dementia of the Alzheimer's Type." *Topics in Geriatric Rehabilitation* 14: 56–75.
Orange, Joseph B., Rosemary B. Lubinski, and D. Jeffery Higginbotham. 1996. "Conversational Repair by Individuals with Dementia of the Alzheimer's Type." *Journal of Speech and Hearing Research* 39: 881–895.
Pajo, Kati. "The Occurrence of 'What,' 'Where,' 'What House' and Other Repair Initiations in the Home Environment of Hearing-impaired Individuals." *International Journal of Language & Communication Disorders* 48 (1): 66–77.
Perkins, Michael R. 2007. *Pragmatic Impairment*. Cambridge: Cambridge University Press.
Perkins, Michael R. 2008. "Pragmatic Impairment As an Emergent Phenomenon." In *The Handbook of Clinical Linguistics*, edited by Martin J. Ball, Michael R. Perkins, Nicole Müller, and Sara Howard. Malden, MA: Blackwell Publishing.
Pomerantz, Anita. 1984. "Agreeing and Disagreeing with Assessments: Some Features of Preferred/Dispreferred Turn Shapes." In *Structures of Social Action*, edited by J. Maxwell Atkinson and John Heritage. Cambridge: Cambridge University Press.
Rapp, Alexander M., and Barbara Wild. 2011. "Nonliteral Language in Alzheimer Dementia: A Review." *Journal of the International Neuropsychological Society* 17 (2): 207–218.
Ridell, Karin. 2008. *Dansk-svenska samtal i praktiken. Språklig interaktion och ackommodation mellan äldre och vårdpersonal i Öresundsregionen* [Danish–Swedish Interaction in Practice: Linguistic Interaction and Accommodation Between the Elderly and Their Caregivers in the Öresund Region]. Uppsala: Uppsala University.
Sarangi, Srikant. 2008. "Editorial." *Communication & Medicine* 5 (1): 2.
Schegloff, Emanuel A. 1987. "Some Sources of Misunderstanding in Talk-in-Interaction." *Linguistics* 25: 201–218.
Schegloff, Emanuel A. 2000. "When 'Others' Initiate Repair." *Applied Linguistics* 21 (2): 205–243.
Schegloff, Emanuel A., Gail Jefferson, and Harvey Sacks. 1977. "The Preference for Self-Correction in the Organization of Repair in Conversation." *Language* 53 (2): 361–382.
Selting, Margret. 1996. "Prosody As an Activity-type Distinctive Cue in Conversation: The Case of So-called 'Astonished' Questions in Repair Initiation." In *Prosody in Conversation*, edited by Elizabeth Couper-Kuhlen and Margret Selting. Cambridge: Cambridge University Press.
Sidnell, Jack. 2012. "The 'Architecture of Intersubjectivity' Revisited: Questions of Species-Uniqueness and Cross-cultural Diversity." Presentation at kick-off seminar for the Finnish Centre of Excellence in Research on Intersubjectivity in Interaction, Helsinki, June 7–9.
Watson, Caroline M., Helen J. Chenery, and Michelle S. Carter. 1999. "An Analysis of Trouble and Repair in the Natural Conversations of People with Dementia of the Alzheimer's Type." *Aphasiology* 13 (5): 195–218.
Wilkinson, Ray. 2007. "Managing Linguistic Incompetence As a Delicate Issue in Aphasic Talk-in-Interaction: On the Use of Laughter in Prolonged Repair Sequences." *Journal of Pragmatics* 39: 542–569.
Wray, Alison. 2008. *Formulaic Language: Pushing the Boundaries*. Oxford: Oxford University Press.

11

"Familyhood" and Young-onset Dementia: Using Narrative and Biography to Understand Longitudinal Adjustment to Diagnosis

PAMELA ROACH, JOHN KEADY, AND PENNY BEE

Introduction

This chapter describes a narrative approach taken to co-construct family biographies with families living with young-onset dementia and discusses how this approach, coupled with a deeper understanding of families' experiences, can contribute to high-quality dementia care and support families in moving beyond the feelings of loss and grief that so often accompany a diagnosis of young-onset dementia. The content of this chapter is based upon a longitudinal, narrative study that gained an in-depth understanding of the day-to-day experience of young-onset dementia in a family-centered context through the use, application, and co-construction of a family biography. The authors worked alongside five younger people with dementia and their nominated family members over a 12–15 month period. In-depth interviews with these family groups were completed alongside the co-construction of family biographies with each family. The co-construction of these biographies acted as a tool to fully involve participating families in the presentation of their narrative story and largely took the form of written stories from families accompanied by personal photographs. Prior to this study, no narrative studies have moved beyond a dyadic model of relationships in order to construct a holistic family narrative that encompasses the experiences of multiple family members and intergenerational dynamics in young-onset dementia (Roach 2010). We begin by outlining the classification and context of young-onset dementia to set this new contribution in context.

Young-onset Dementia: Classification and Context

Young-onset dementia (dementia occurring younger than the age of sixty-five) has been shown to have a myriad of social and personal effects on every individual within a family system. Critical factors, such as age, employability, family composition, and presentation of dementia symptoms can create intensified experiences and increased stress for younger people with dementia and their families (Brown and Roach 2010; Page and Keady 2010; Svanberg, Stott, and Spector 2010; Roach et al. 2008; Beattie et al. 2004; Harris 2004; Williams, Dearden, and Cameron 2001). In a previously published literature review (Roach et al. 2008), loss and grief emerged as aspects of the relational experience of dementia where additional support was needed by younger people and their families in order to live positively with a diagnosis of dementia. This relational aspect of care is often lacking from dementia care services (Roach et al. 2008).

Despite such an acknowledgement there remains a paucity of published literature in the dementia field that strives to work in a family-centered way. Those studies that have aimed to include family members often exclude the person with dementia from their definition of the "family" unit (Garwick, Detzner, and Boss 1994). This type of approach serves to silence the voice of the person with dementia and locates them outside the family unit. Other studies have included family members of people with dementia as participants but typically do so largely with the aim of constructing a narrative of the person with dementia's life and experience, not as active contributors to their own family group (Crichton and Koch 2007). Although study designs may be inclusive in the way they allow the person with dementia to narrate their own story and include the views of a family member (Koch and Crichton 2007), they are rarely concerned with the family life story as a whole and thus may actually fail to represent a holistic family-centered view of the experience of young-onset dementia. Work with older adults has aimed to recruit families in order to examine how these family structures may best support the person with dementia in a meaningful way but primarily only examine the dyadic experience between two individuals, even where the original stated aim was to explore a "shared" family experience (Kellett et al. 2010; Phinney 2006).

A recent review of dementia caregiving in spousal relationships confirms this prevailing dyadic perspective (Braun et al. 2009). It is unclear why dyads, and particularly spousal dyads, remain the primary unit of "family experience" explored in dementia research, given that families have long been acknowledged to substantially influence the quality of care that a person with dementia receives at home and in that way to influence their health-related quality of life (Adams 1987). Family members do not exist in isolation from one another; they have a shared history, a shared future, and often a shared biology. Individual views and experiences are shaped by being part of this group (Copeland and White 1991) and the memories, stories, and narratives that are shared by this group may vary according to the way that they are constructed by individuals (Roberts 2002). To date, however, little research has been done to examine the experience of dementia from a family perspective and no work to date has specifically explored the family experience of young-onset dementia. Arguably it is this added family dimension that needs to be considered when working clinically with younger people with dementia and their families in order to allow the family unit to move beyond loss and live and work together with a diagnosis of young-onset dementia.

Service Delivery and Organization

Specialist young-onset services are recommended as "best practice" for younger people with dementia but policy guidance as to how these services should be configured remains unclear. The literature suggests that where these services do exist they are often inadequate and in many cases the opinions of younger people with dementia are not considered in service design. Moreover, where specific services for younger people do not exist, younger people are often referred to older people's services. As a result, some will question the appropriateness of these clinical services; others will dismiss older people's services altogether, thus leaving them without specialist dementia care of any kind. Their own needs and the needs of their families then remain unmet (Beattie et al. 2004; Beattie et al. 2002). The literature recommends that assessment and care planning should consider age-appropriate environments by providing information to maintain the individuality of the younger person with dementia. Due to the complexity of the intergenerational relationships often present in these cases, it is crucial that family-centered care is integrated into any new specialist care structure and services should consider the needs and experiences of social networks, including family, friends, and work colleagues when working with younger people with dementia (Keady and Matthew 1997). A sense of loss and the ability to move on from a diagnosis of young-onset dementia in order to live positively as a family have been previously reported as important aspects to the family experience of young-onset dementia (Roach et al. 2008) and it is this that became a key focus of the authors' work.

Using Family Relationships and Narrative Biography to Enhance Clinical Practice

The narrative family biography describes how families live in the present day with young-onset dementia and how as a family unit they may be influenced by a dominant family storyline that predates any diagnosis of young-onset dementia. This approach necessitates the collection of biographical information from families in order to understand how they may use or respond to their dominant storylines and how this may in turn affect their clinical support needs. The use of varying storylines and their impact on families can influence periods of positive or negative coping, in turn highlighting times of increased need from services. Understanding family biography may simplify some of the complex family relationships that clinicians struggle to address in a relational capacity, enhancing family understanding and potentially facilitating a way for family-centered care to be integrated into clinical services.

The work presented in this chapter reflects and enhances prior research into family systems and chronic illness (Rolland 1994; Rolland 1988). However, this chapter acknowledges a more dynamic relationship between family functioning and the experience of a chronic condition, whereby family functioning affects the experience of living with a condition but the experience of living with that condition can also have a great impact on family functioning. This interdependence between the experience of young-onset dementia and family functioning will be grounded in the biographical family narrative of individual family units.

The family-centered approach described here elevates the status of the family in order to address the potential loss of a family's sense of self via transitions in the family biography. Loss of self has been addressed previously in the literature in dementia (Sabat 2002), but also within the broader context of chronic illness (Charmaz 2002; Charmaz 1983). Recognizing that families may be in danger of losing their constructed unit's sense of selfhood, or "familyhood," as a direct result of a condition such as young-onset dementia provides substantial motivation to more fully integrate family-centered care into professional working practices. Using biographical knowledge collected through narrative methods can help clinical staff to guide families through transitions, such as the loss of the ability to drive or a move to a long-term care facility. It moves families beyond this potential sense of loss, enabling them to continue to function as a family unit based on their historical dominant family storyline.

Previous work has not only demonstrated the value of life-story and biography work in clinical dementia settings (Keady, Williams, and Hughes-Roberts 2005), but also that practice development based on the experiences of people with dementia is essential to providing person-centered care (Keady,

Williams, and Hughes-Roberts 2005). Although this study argues the case for a more family-centered approach to young-onset dementia care, the principles of practice development remain the same. Effective practice development is just one of a number of issues to be addressed when considering the potential advantages and limitations to the implementation of biographical, family-centered care to clinical practice. There may be identifiable barriers to family-centered care presented from service-providers, policy-makers, and service-users; it is not only identifying but also challenging these barriers and recognizing the advantages of working with families holistically that can move the traditionally held dyadic approach to family care to a truly family-centered way of working.

Defining Family

One barrier the authors are trying to address in their work is the definition of "family." The term "family" in the literature in dementia has also become synonymous with the term "carer" (Braun et al. 2009). The literature base is clear in its reference to "family carers" (Papastavrou et al. 2007; Brodaty, Green, and Koschera 2003; Freyne et al. 1999; Pearlin et al. 1990) and UK policy uses the terms "family" and "carer" interchangeably in reference to a primary significant other who is expected to take on caring responsibilities for the person with dementia (Department of Health 2009; National Institute for Health and Clinical Excellence and Social Care Institute for Excellence 2006; Department of Health 2005; Department of Health 2001a; Department of Health 1999). Not only will this affect the person with dementia's sense of self by changing them into a "sufferer" and altering how they are seen by others (Sabat 2002), but it may also alter the family member's sense of self by moving their role from a familial to a caring context. The study reported herein aimed to move the younger person with dementia back into their family unit, a place that they have traditionally had to abandon within the published dementia "family" literature (Braun et al. 2009; Crichton and Koch 2007; Garwick, Detzner, and Boss 1994) and by doing so providing a safeguard against the potential threat of loss of "familyhood." Throughout the study families operated as units based on their historical relationships and have been treated as such. Families in this context were defined as:

> a social context of two or more people characterized by mutual attachment, caring, long-term commitment, and responsibility to provide individual growth, supportive relationships, health of members and

of the unit, and maintenance of the organization and system during constant individual, family and societal change. (Craft and Willadsen 1992, 519)

Accordingly, the term "family" was used to denote any and all members of a family configuration; a configuration determined by the younger person with dementia and the significant others in their life, be they biologically related or not. These significant others are not labeled as "carers" and there was a purposeful lack of focus on the burden or suffering they may have faced as separate entities to the person with dementia. This topic has been explored frequently in previous literature (Papastavrou et al. 2007; Shaji et al. 2003; Freyne et al. 1999; Carlson and Robertson 1993; Pearlin et al. 1990). Rather, the focus remains firmly on the shared day-to-day experience of living with a diagnosis of young-onset dementia as a family.

In addition to defining "family" in a clinical care context, a related potential complicating factor in the successful implementation of family-centered care is the cooperation of families themselves. For some families experiencing young-onset dementia, there are historical issues that may prevent them from fully participating as a family unit based on their biographical family functioning. However, as clinical care culture perceptions of what constitutes family care and how families are defined change, this shift in paradigm may be reflected by service users and they may begin to conceptualize the holistic family unit as the unit of therapeutic engagement. The prospect of changing the definition of "family" when working with younger people with dementia has implications for the way in which care is provided and may require staff to approach relational aspects of care in a more in-depth manner than previously considered (Roach et al. 2008).

Improving Nursing Practice through Family-based Care

Improving this relational care in nursing practice has been addressed previously in the literature where Liaschenko and Fisher (1999) have described a theory of understanding how relational care fits into current care provision. The authors outline a framework of different levels of "knowledge" in nursing practice. These levels of knowledge are (1) "case," knowledge of the physiological and disease processes; (2) "patient," knowledge of response to treatment and movement through the health and social care system; (3) "person," knowledge of an individual's personal biography; and (4) "relational," the knowledge of how case, patient, and person knowledge are linked to and influence the other (Liaschenko and Fisher 1999). This form of knowledge acknowledges the "patient" as the owner of their own biography and as experts in the condition (Nolan et al. 2007; Keady et al. 2007). This is now reflected in health care practice with the advent of the "expert patient" (Department of Health 2001b) and increasing recognition of the value of service users and families contributing their "voice" to health care provision (NHS 2010); facilitated further by the creation of open forums for patient experiences (see http://www.patientopinion.org.uk/). The extension of the "person" knowledge to "family" knowledge via family biography is at the core of providing family-centered care and encouraging staff to use their relational skills and personal knowledge of their care recipients to enhance their clinical decision-making (Keady et al. 2007), empowering both staff and care recipients (be this individual or family).

Additionally, it has now long been recognized that people with dementia live with their condition in a social context with those around them (Sabat 2002; Downs 2000). Adequate training for clinical staff, as well as appropriate support from care managers and health and social care policy makers is necessary to encourage staff to undertake an inclusive and family-centered approach to work with younger people with dementia that fully acknowledges the value of this personal/family and relational knowledge. To continue to limit care provision based on narrow definitions of family and related knowledge of their patients means that younger people with dementia and their families will not be in receipt of a biopsychosocial model of dementia care (National Institute for Health and Clinical Excellence and Social Care Institute for Excellence 2006). As such, their quality of life may be adversely affected.

Despite current barriers, a family-centered approach has distinct advantages when working with younger people with dementia due to the potential of increased complexity of intergenerational family dynamics and increased family distress in young-onset dementia (Harris and Keady 2009; Roach et al. 2008; Tindall and Manthorpe 1997). A greater understanding of the family experience, potential trajectory of family functioning, and relational issues between family members may provide valuable insight into the true impact of young-onset dementia on a family unit. It has been shown in the family caregiving literature that family relationships impact the efficacy of interventions (Luscombe, Brodaty, and Freeth 1998; Schumacher, Stewart, and Archbold 1998; Fisher and Lieberman 1994) and are influenced by a family's transgenerational history of illness and belief systems (Rolland 1988). An in-depth understanding of the family's biography and functioning may aid clinicians in their decision-making to provide high-quality care to younger people with dementia and their families.

Integrating a Family-centered Biographical Approach in Research

This chapter has briefly considered the definition of family and the likely value of family-based care to clinical service and nursing practice. In the remainder of the chapter we outline a longitudinal, narrative study undertaken with the primary aim of locating younger people with dementia within their construction of a family, with their role in that family integral to the research design and act, thus adhering to the family-centered approach described above.

Younger people with dementia were the first individuals of any family recruited into the study through clinical services so that their central position in the family and control over potential participants was maintained. The younger person with dementia was then free to nominate up to five "family members" for participation (Roach 2010). Empowering the younger person with dementia to have control over who is included in the construction of the family unit ensures that they remain central to their dementia "story" and that the family's biography is centered on the younger person with dementia. Empowering and supporting younger people with dementia to define their family is a methodological technique that has been partially undertaken in previous studies working with people with mental illness where family members are defined by primary caregivers (Tweedell et al. 2004; Garwick, Detzner, and Boss 1994). This study is unique in the way that the definition of "family" is left firmly in the hands of the person with dementia. This actively involves and empowers people with dementia by providing choices, as recommended in the literature (Cayton 2004; Wilkinson 2002).

Five families were recruited from a variety of specialist young-onset and non-specialist clinical dementia services in the northwest of England and participated in the study for a period between twelve and fifteen months each. The mean age of younger people with dementia upon entry to the study was fifty-nine years of age ($sd = 5.79$), with the mean age at diagnosis being fifty-seven years ($sd = 7.11$). The time stated by the families between the first noticeable signs of (undiagnosed) young-onset dementia and receiving a diagnosis ranged from between six and fifteen months, with the mean being slightly over eleven months ($sd = 3.29$). The sample comprised two men and three women. All had already retired or ceased working at entry to the study; three of the five had retired or ceased working prior to receiving a diagnosis; the other two had been in employment when initially presenting with symptoms but had ceased working around the time of diagnosis. The mean age of participating family members at entry into the study was fifty-eight years ($sd = 15.00$), the range was 32–76 years. The mean time known to the younger person with dementia was 35.50 years ($sd = 17.16$)

and the range was 12–64 years. Every younger person with dementia requested their spouse's participation. Three of the families consisted of only this spousal dyad. One other family consisted of the younger person with dementia, her current husband, and her daughter from a previous marriage; the fifth family included the younger person with dementia, her husband, her uncle, and her younger brother.

Data were collected by co-constructing family biographies and using in-depth interviewing to collect rich data on the experience of family adjustment, coping, and decision-making. Biographical working provided a nonthreatening method of data collection that enabled families to retain control over their "story" while providing rich description of their experiences. It also provided a way for the researcher to access and understand the holistic experiences of participating families prior to and following on from a diagnosis of young-onset dementia. This avoided defining the family members by such a diagnosis, and recognized the significance of their long-standing familial relationships and dynamics.

Building Relationships and Biographical Working with Families

Developing relationships and building trust with families is as important when conducting research with people with dementia and their families as it is when interacting clinically (Nygård 2006). Interviews were conducted collectively with each of the family groups and although there were opportunities provided for individual interviews, it was rare that this was requested by any family member. All interviews took place at the home of one member of the family. Arrangements were also made for families (including the younger person with dementia) to have telephone and email contact with the researcher between visits if they felt there were any issues or biographical themes they needed to discuss. Families were encouraged to bring their own materials (photographs, stories, physical objects, and so on) to prompt memories and encourage discussion. It is preferable to be in surroundings familiar to the participants and ideally in their own home when constructing biographies in this way so that they feel relaxed, and precious objects, photographs, and mementos can be integrated into the research contact (Wicks and Whiteford 2006). These items can also stimulate stories and conversation (Roberts 2002) and help to keep the data collection and interviews flexible so that it remains as accessible and inclusive as possible for the person with dementia (Nygård 2006).

As a way to structure such interviews, the process used in the study that forms the basis for this chapter may provide a useful starting point. The first visit with each family was an in-depth, semistructured interview to uncover themes and "chapters" to discuss in relation to the family biography at later visits. The primary question at the first interview was, "If you were to write a book about your family, what do you think the chapters might be called?" The possible chapter titles of the family biography were used flexibly as a base for the interviews undertaken in following visits. Further details specific to the frequency and duration of the visits and interviews with each family are reported elsewhere (Roach 2010). Alternative methods of data collection (drawing, video diaries, and so on) were discussed with families and all families were provided with empty scrapbooks and the materials with which to create their family biographies within these books. These materials included pens, glue, tape, pencils, and cameras. Examples of family trees and a set of instructions formatted as a "helpful hint and tip" sheet were also provided to help families initially "get started" with the co-construction of their family biographies. The hint and tip sheet included such items such as drawing a family tree, chaptering their lives as a family, outlining the "major" events in their shared experience, and asking them to discuss with one another what they considered to be important topics for inclusion in their biography (i.e., pets, holidays, family gatherings or events). These activities can provide researchers and/or care providers with information crucial to understanding the functioning of individual family units.

This co-construction of family biographies comprised the primary objective of the reported study and was undertaken in a collaborative way while being participant-led by the families as much as possible. Each family conceptualized their family through a unique lens and, indeed, constructed their family biography in these individualized ways. The duration of contact with participating families allowed both parties to gain trust from one another and become comfortable with what was a novel and creative process. Most of the families required more direction than had been anticipated by the researcher and the early attempts at family biography co-construction became very much a shared experience. When families reached a level of comfort with what they felt was "expected" of them they demonstrated an increased sense of ownership over their biographies, and more easily took control of the co-construction of them.

Families were encouraged to think about the meanings and significance of what they were including in each of their family biographies. This meant that they often were asked to think about times in their life or feelings for each other that had previously been left unexplored. While some families found this difficult, all families reported at the end of the study that they found participating to be a helpful and enjoyable experience. The building of relationships that made up a large part of the initial interviews with all the families allowed for these difficult subjects to be explored and discussed in detail and this was as much a part of the process as the physical construction of the biographical "books." Thus, the establishment of a trusting relationship is vital to gaining an in-depth understanding of the experiences of family units living with young-onset dementia.

Although not all family members identified as integral to the functioning of each family unit participated in the study, these key family members were present in the discussions and the co-construction of the biographies, illustrating the inherent complexity and interdependency present in family networks. The development of an in-depth understanding of these complex relationships and how these relationships influence the experience of young-onset dementia and efficacy of clinical interventions is crucial to developing high-quality, needs-based dementia care for families living with a diagnosis of young-onset dementia. Understanding the sense of loss and the importance of moving forward in the historical familial context is integral to providing this high-quality, needs-based care.

Understanding Adjustment and the Family Experience through Biography

Narratives, and therefore family biographies, are "personal accounts of people's motives, experiences and actions and the way they interpret and assign meaning to them" (Holloway and Freshwater 2007, 5), and it is thus the family biography and "storyline" that become the objects of analysis. Ongoing narrative analysis of the family biographies was undertaken contemporaneously throughout the period of data collection using holistic narrative analysis (Lieblich, Tuval-Mashiach, and Zilber 1998; Riessman 1993) of each family's interview data and categorical content analysis (Riessman 1993) of overarching themes, as well as a structured narrative analysis of included photographs (Riessman 2008; Banks 2007). Further details of the process of analysis are reported and can be found elsewhere (Roach 2010). As the research relationships continued with the participating families, clarification of the author's interpretations about interview or visual data was sought and developing themes of narrative analysis were discussed. Through this ongoing analysis of the individual family biographies, the dominant family storyline of each family emerged. A dominant family storyline is typically grounded in the individual family biography and based on (1) shared expectations, of each other and the future; (2) continuity, their future family storyline aligned with their dominant biographical family storyline; and (3) their relationships with one another. By extending the narrative analysis of the data across the family biographies (Riessman 2008; Banks 2007; Lieblich Tuval-Mashiach, and Zilber 1998; Riessman 1993), and cognizant of the dominant family storylines of each case, five transcending storyline types emerged as ways in which families adjusted to and lived with their experience of young-onset dementia. Presented alphabetically, the identified storyline types were as follows:

1. Agreeing: An agreeing storyline refers to a narrative discourse presented "as one," where role boundaries are negotiated and understood and a strong shared narrative line of "togetherness" is evident. Agreeing storylines were used to maintain openness in the family unit and to share experiences with one another and was the most open and positive family storyline found in the data. From the five case studies, this openness and sharing of experiences took place when there had been transparency to the family relationships that predated the diagnosis of young-onset dementia.
2. Colluding: Colluding storylines were seen in the data when two or more family members "colluded with one another" in order to maintain a storyline that was important to family functioning in some way. This may mean that the younger person with dementia is colluding with some (but not necessarily all) of their family members, or that some family members are colluding separately from the younger person with dementia. Inherent in this storyline is the idea that not all family members are working toward the same shared/agreed storyline and that there is some dissonance between the experiences of young-onset dementia of the "colluding individuals" versus "noncolluding individuals," thus "closing off" part of the family. This has the potential to negatively affect the sense of self of a younger person with dementia by altering the way they are viewed by others and the way they view themselves in relation to such individuals (Sabat 2002; Kitwood 1997).
3. Conflicting: A conflicting storyline represents disagreement and divergence in presentation and may represent areas of hostility. Family members using conflicting storylines may take on active roles in the provocation of others, which may detrimentally influence the long-term sense of self of all those involved thereby altering internal and external perceptions of one another (Sabat 2002).
4. Fabricating: Fabricating storylines are consciously used to alter details to fit into a conceptualization of the "truth" and "family." This storyline type can be used to mislead and misinform whether consciously or otherwise.
5. Protecting: Protecting storylines can be used to ameliorate stress and identity within the family relationships and have the potential to be disempowering to younger people with dementia or other family members. Protecting storylines were also seen to be used as a method of adjustment to the new diagnosis and balance within the family.

The specific ways in which these storyline types were generated and used by the families in this study, and how they may influence the family experience of young-onset dementia are reported elsewhere (Roach 2010) as the focus of this chapter remains on the implications and integration of family biography to current dementia care practice and research.

Implications for Dementia Care Practice

Families are complex entities and are integral to the experience of living with young-onset dementia. The younger person with dementia is part of a "dominant family storyline" and this storyline affects how a family unit copes and adjusts to transitions in their experience. It would appear essential to adopt a family-centered approach in order to enhance young-onset dementia care provision. In order to do this, it is necessary to understand how the individual biography of families impacts upon the storylines used by family members to cope with and adapt to a diagnosis of young-onset dementia. It is understandable that the longitudinal and in-depth approach taken in this study may not be feasible for many care providers to implement in the same manner. There are, however, a series of mechanisms and recommendations that can easily be integrated into clinical dementia care.

First, it is crucial to learn who the family members are and what their roles are in the family structure. This includes not only biologically related individuals but any significant other as identified by the younger person with dementia and their families. Second, it is vital to record or plot biographical data. To understand how a family unit functions, it is necessary to have an understanding about how their life as a family unit has progressed and the experiences they have shared as a family. This frames their experience and influences the types of storylines employed throughout the lived experience. Understanding and plotting the family biography also enables understanding about how and why families function in different ways. This may be done in various ways and does not have to be conceptualized as the "books" were in this study. Simple timeline charts or notes that can be kept with the patient record are techniques that are both time-efficient for staff and meaningful for service users. Such timelines could be simplified by using important "major" life events as starting points (births, deaths, marriages, and so forth) before the addition of important milestones for each individual family. Third, clinical care providers need to invest in families. Long-term commitment of repeated visits and continued interest in families' lives is necessary in order to establish family functioning and move beyond the public narrative created for the consumption of health and social care professionals. This does not need to significantly impact staff time or health care resources. This type of investment in the family biography is an activity that may be done by any staff member in regular contact with people with dementia and their families. In the reported study it was apparent that this repeated and prolonged contact was made by all clinical staff, regardless of role, it was just that the collection and collation of the "family story" was not a primary clinical concern. Fourth, an inclusive definition of family is needed in order to gain insight from all family perspectives by engaging more than the primary caregiver. Traditionally, family members have been viewed as separate and distinct units to the person with dementia; young-onset dementia is no different, and the term "family" has implied "primary caregiver." These restricted perceptions of "family" do not provide a complete understanding of the interpersonal dynamics at work within family networks. A new, family-centered and inclusive view of "family" in dementia care is needed that locates the person with dementia within their family unit and their historical familial role. The inclusion of additional family members in care provision and care planning is likely to be one key way to achieve this family-centered structure. Finally, family-centered care can only be fully integrated if family biography is used to inform clinical decision-making. Family biographical data may provide a useful starting point for clinical staff to simplify complex family relationships and move relational aspects of service provision from the social realm into the professional realm in a way in which they feel confident in providing treatment, intervention, and information based on individual family relationships.

Through working with families in this way, clinical practice can be enhanced to take into account not only the individual biography of a family, but their relational support needs through times of transition. In some ways relationship-centered care aims to include this aspect of support but focuses primarily on relationships between service users and professional carers and separates the person with dementia from their carer (Nolan et al. 2006; Beach et al. 2006; Nolan, Keady, and Aveyard 2001; Tresolini and The Pew-Fetzer Task Force 1994). Family relationships are attended to in the relationship-centered care model, but again, in a family "carer" context rather than a family "member" context (Beach et al. 2006; Tresolini and The Pew-Fetzer Task Force 1994). Although an important advancement of relationship-centered care is to recognize that all therapeutic exchanges exist within a relational context (Ryan et al. 2008; Beach et al. 2006; Nolan, Keady, and Aveyard 2001; Tresolini and The Pew-Fetzer Task Force 1994), a family-centered paradigm recognizes that relationships exist and influence care outside of these formal therapeutic exchanges. Family biography is one method of capturing these relationships within clinical settings. The work completed in this study and the concepts developed were supported by local practitioners when shared after project completion and would benefit from further clinical and empirical testing. In order to facilitate change within practice, it is crucial to work closely with clinical staff in order to encourage reflective and evidence-based practice based on the needs of their service users and their families. Future research needs to encourage families to participate as groups, to empower all family members to realize their contribution to the family unit's functioning is valuable and that they have needs to be addressed by clinical services. In this way clinical staff working with younger people with dementia and their families can use biographical data and family storylines informed by the narrative methods outlined here to enhance clinical care provision. This may provide families with new ways to live positively within the context of their historical family context and move beyond the loss experienced during times of transition (Roach et al. 2008) through appropriate and individualized family-centered care provision.

References

Adams, Trevor. 1987. "Dementia Is a Family Affair." *Community Outlook*, February, 7–9.
Banks, Marcus. 2007. *Using Visual Data in Qualitative Research*. London: Sage.
Beach, Mary Catherine, Thomas Inui, and Relationship-Centered Care Research Network. 2006. "Relationship-Centered Care: A Constructive Reframing." *Journal of General Internal Medicine* 21: S3-S8.
Beattie, Angela, Gavin Daker-White, Jane Gilliard, and Robin Means. 2002. "Younger People in Dementia Care: A Review of Service Needs, Service Provision and Models of Good Practice." *Aging and Mental Health* 6: 205–212.
Beattie, Angela, Gavin Daker-White, Jane Gilliard, and Robin Means. 2004. "'How Can They Tell?' A Qualitative Study of the Views of Younger People about their Dementia and Dementia Care Services." *Health and Social Care in the Community* 12: 359–368.
Braun, Melanie, Urte Scholz, Barbara Bailey, Sonja Perren, Ranier Hornung, and Mike Martin. 2009. "Dementia Caregiving in Spousal Relationships: A Dyadic Perspective." *Aging and Mental Health* 13: 426–436.
Brodaty, Henry, Alisa Green, and Annette Koschera. 2003. "Meta-Analysis of Psychosocial Interventions for Caregivers of People with Dementia." *Journal of the American Geriatrics Society* 51: 657–664.
Brown, Anne, and Pamela Roach. 2010. "My Husband has Young-onset Dementia: A Daughter, Wife and Mother's Story." *Dementia* 9: 451.
Carlson, Keith, and Sharon Robertson. 1993. "Husbands and Wives of Dementia Patients: Burden and Social Support." *Canadian Journal of Rehabilitation* 6: 163–173.
Cayton, Harry. 2004. "Telling Stories: Choices and Challenges on the Journey of Dementia." *Dementia* 3: 9–17.
Charmaz, Kathy. 1983. "Loss of Self: A Fundamental Form of Suffering in the Chronically Ill." *Sociology of Health and Illness* 5: 168–195.
Charmaz, Kathy. 2002. "Stories and Silences: Disclosures and Self in Chronic Illness." *Qualitative Inquiry* 8: 302–328.
Copeland, Anne, and Kathleen White. 1991. *Studying Families*. Newbury Park: SAGE Publications.
Craft, Martha, and Jennifer Willadsen. 1992. "Interventions Related to Family." *Nursing Clinics of North America* 27: 517–540.
Crichton, Jonathan, and Tina Koch. 2007. "Living with Dementia: Curating Self-identity." *Dementia* 6: 365–381.

Department of Health. 1999. *Caring about Carers: A National Strategy for Carers*. London: Department of Health.
Department of Health. 2001a. *National Service Framework for Older People*. London: Department of Health.
Department of Health. 2001b. *The Expert Patient: A New Approach to Chronic Disease Management in the 21st Century*. London: Department of Health.
Department of Health. 2005. *Everybody's Business. Integrated Mental Health Services for Older Adults: A Service Development Guide*. London: Department of Health.
Department of Health. 2009. *Living Well With Dementia: A National Dementia Strategy*. London: Department of Health.
Downs, Murna. 2000. "Dementia in a Socio-cultural Context: An Idea Whose Time has Come." *Ageing and Society* 20: 369–375.
Fisher, Lawrence, and Morton Lieberman. 1994. "Alzheimer's Disease: The Impact of the Family on Spouses, Offspring, and Inlaws." *Family Process* 33: 305–325.
Freyne, Aideen, Nick Kidd, Robert Coen, and Brian Lawlor. 1999. "Burden in Carers of Dementia Patients: Higher Levels in Carers of Younger Sufferers." *International Journal of Geriatric Psychiatry* 14: 784–788.
Garwick, Ann, Daniel Detzner, Pauline Boss. 1994. "Family Perceptions of Living with Alzheimer's Disease." *Family Process* 33: 327–340.
Harris, Phyllis Braudy. 2004. "The Perspective of Younger People with Dementia: Still an Overlooked Population." *Social Work in Mental Health* 2: 17–36.
Harris, Phyllis Braudy, and John Keady. 2009. "Selfhood in Younger Onset Dementia: Transitions and Testimonies." *Aging and Mental Health* 13: 437–444.
Holloway, Immy, and Dawn Freshwater. 2007. *Narrative Research in Nursing*. Oxford: Blackwell.
Keady, John, Susan Ashcroft-Simpson, Kath Halligan, Sion Williams. 2007. "Admiral Nursing and the Family Care of a Parent with Dementia: Using Autobiographical Narrative as Grounding for Negotiated Clinical Practice and Decision-making." *Scandinavian Journal of Caring Science* 21: 345–353.
Keady, John, and Liz Matthew. 1997. "Younger People with Dementia." *Elderly Care* 9: 19–23.
Keady, John, Sion Williams, and John Hughes-Roberts. 2005. "Emancipatory Practice Development through Life-story Work: Changing Care in a Memory Clinic in North Wales." *Practice Development in Health Care* 4: 203–212.
Kellett, Ursula, Wendy Moyle, Margaret McAllister, Christopher King, and Fran Gallagher. 2010. "Life Stories and Biography: A Means of Connecting Family and Staff to People with Dementia." *Journal of Clinical Nursing* 19: 1707–1715.
Kitwood, Tom. 1997. *Dementia Reconsidered: The Person Comes First*. Buckingham: Open University Press.
Koch, Tina, and Jonathan Crichton. 2007. "Innovative Approaches to Living with Dementia: An Australian Case Study." In *User Participation in Health and Social Care Research: Voices, Values and Evaluation*, edited by Mike Nolan, Elizabeth Hanson, Gordon Grant and John Keady. Maidenhead: Open University Press.
Liaschenko, Joan, and Anastasia Fisher. 1999. "Theorizing the Knowledge that Nurses Use in the Conduct of their Work." *Scholarly Inquiry for Nursing Practice* 13: 29–41.
Lieblich, Amia, Rivka Tuval-Mashiach, and Tamar Zilber. 1998. *Narrative Research: Reading, Analysis and Interpretation*. London: Sage.
Luscombe, Georgina, Henry Brodaty, and Stephen Freeth. 1998. "Younger People with Dementia: Diagnostic Issues, Effects on Carers and Use of Services." *International Journal of Geriatric Psychiatry* 13: 323–330.
National Health Service. 2010. Patient Opinion. National Health Service [On-line]. http://www.patientopinion.org.uk/. Accessed 23 August 2012.
National Institute for Health and Clinical Excellence and Social Care Institute for Excellence. 2006. *NICE Clinical Guideline 42. Dementia: Supporting People with Dementia and their Careers in Health and Social Care*. London: NICE.

Nolan, Mike, Jayne Brown, Sue Davies, Janet Nolan, and John Keady. 2006. *The Senses Framework: Improving Care for Older People Through a Relationship-Centred Approach. GRIP Report Number 2.* Sheffield: University of Sheffield.

Nolan, Mike, Elizabeth Hanson, Gordon Grant, John Keady, and Lennart Magnusson. 2007. "Introduction: What Counts as Knowledge, Whose Knowledge Counts? Towards Authentic Participatory Enquiry." In *User Participation in Health and Social Care Research,* edited by Mike Nolan, Elizabeth Hanson, Gordon Grant and John Keady. Maidenhead: Open University Press.

Nolan, Mike, John Keady, and Barry Aveyard. 2001. "Relationship-centred Care Is the Next Logical Step." *British Journal of Nursing* 10: 757.

Nygård, Louise. 2006. "How Can We Get Access to the Experiences of People with Dementia? Suggestions and Reflections." *Scandinavian Journal of Occupational Therapy* 13: 101–112.

Page, Sean, and John Keady. 2010. "Sharing Stories: A Meta-ethnographic Analysis of 12 Autobiographies Written by People with Dementia between 1989 and 2007." *Ageing and Society* 30: 511–526.

Papastavrou, Evridiki, Athena Kalokerinou, Savvas Papacostas, Haritini Tsangari, and Panagiota Sourtzi. 2007. "Caring for a Relative with Dementia: Family Caregiver Burden." *Journal of Advanced Nursing* 58: 446–457.

Pearlin, Leonard, Joseph Mullan, Shirley Semple, and Marilyn Skaff. 1990. "Caregiving and the Stress Process: An Overview of Concepts and Their Measures." *The Gerontologist* 30: 583–594.

Phinney, Alison. 2006. "Family Strategies for Supporting Involvement in Meaningful Activity by Persons with Dementia." *Journal of Family Nursing* 12: 80–101.

Riessman, Catherine Kohler. 1993. *Narrative Analysis.* Newbury Park: Sage.

Riessman, Catherine Kohler. 2008. *Narrative Methods for the Human Sciences.* Thousand Oaks: Sage.

Roach, Pamela. 2010. "A Family-Centred Study of Younger People with Dementia." PhD Diss., University of Manchester.

Roach, Pamela, John Keady, Penny Bee, and Kevin Hope. 2008. "Subjective Experiences of Younger People with Dementia and their Families: Implications for UK Research, Policy and Practice." *Reviews in Clinical Gerontology* 18: 165–174.

Roberts, Brian. 2002. *Biographical Research.* Buckingham: Open University Press.

Rolland, John. 1988. "A Conceptual Model of Chronic and Life-Threatening Illness and Its Impact on Families." In *Families in Trouble: Knowledge and Practice Perspectives for Professionals in the Human Services,* edited by C. S. Chilman, F. M. Cox, and E. W. Nunnally. Newbury Park: SAGE.

Rolland, John. 1994. *Families, Illness and Disability. An Integrative Treatment Model.* New York: Basic Books.

Ryan, Tony, Mike Nolan, David Reid, and Pam Enderby. 2008. "Using the Senses Framework to Achieve Relationship-centred Dementia Care Services." *Dementia* 7: 71–93.

Sabat, Steven. 2002. "Surviving Manifestations of Selfhood in Alzheimer's Disease." *Dementia* 1: 25–36.

Schumacher, Karen, Barbara Stewart, and Patricia Archbold. 1998. "Conceptualization and Measurement of Doing Family Caregiving Well." *Journal of Nursing Scholarship* 30: 63–67.

Shaji, K. S., K. Smitha, K. Praveen Lal, and Martin Prince. 2003. "Caregivers of People with Alzheimer's Disease: A Qualitative Study from the Indian 10/66 Dementia Research Network." *International Journal of Geriatric Psychiatry* 18: 1–6.

Svanberg, Emma, Joshua Stott, and Aimee Spector. 2010. "'Just Helping': Children Living with a Parent with Young Onset Dementia." *Aging and Mental Health* 14: 740–751.

Tindall, Linda, and Jill Manthorpe. 1997. "Early Onset Dementia: A Case of Ill-timing?" *Journal of Mental Health* 6: 237–249.

Tresolini, Carol, and The Pew-Fetzer Task Force. 1994. *Health Professions, Education and Relationship-Centered Care.* San Francisco: Pew Health Professions Commission.

Tweedell, Donna, Cheryl Forchuk, Jackie Jewell, and Lianne Steinnagel. 2004. "Families' Experience during Recovery or Nonrecovery from Psychosis." *Archives of Psychiatric Nursing* 18: 17–25.

Wicks, Alison, and Gail Whiteford. 2006. "Conceptual and Practical Issues in Qualitative Research: Reflections on a Life-history Study." *Scandinavian Journal of Occupational Therapy* 13: 94–100.

Wilkinson, Heather. 2002. "Including People with Dementia in Research: Methods and Motivations." In *The Perspectives of People with Dementia: Research Methods and Motivations*, edited by Heather Wilkinson. London: Jessica Kingsley Publishers.

Williams, Tim, Anthony Dearden, and Ian Cameron. 2001. "From Pillar to Post—A Study of Younger People with Dementia." *Psychiatric Bulletin* 25: 384–387.

12

The Subjectivity of Disorientation: Moral Stakes and Concerns

LINDA ÖRULV

Problems of disorientation, in the sense of not knowing where one is, are common in Alzheimer's disease, and increasingly so as the disease progresses. On a social level, disorientation entails uncertainty about general conduct norms. How to behave in a socially acceptable way is highly dependent on where one is and what relation one has to the place. A person has normative bonds to places, including rights and authority, duties and expectations. These are linked to certain positions, such as host or hostess, guest, customer, or resident. For people with Alzheimer's disease in residential care, such bonds and relations are blurred. Unsure of where they are or why they are there, residents are left with little guidance on what to do next, where to go, or what to expect from a situation.

In many cases caregivers are able to establish what seems to be mutual understanding of the situation (Eggers, Norberg, and Ekman 2005; Öhlander 1996; Vittoria 1999), especially as less is expected from persons with dementia. However, not only are such established understandings sometimes subject to negotiation (Öhlander 1996; Diaz Moore 1999), but they also may not always take into account residents' personal stakes and concerns, especially moral ones. This may cause much anxiety for someone who is eager to do her share, pay her way, and not cause anybody inconvenience—to be a morally responsible, decent, and "nice" person. People with Alzheimer's disease have been found to keep their moral values and outlooks on life intact as the disease evolves, and may embrace them as something that matters deeply (Örulv and Hydén 2006; Westius, Andersson, and Kallenberg 2009; Westius, Kallenberg, and Norberg 2010). "[H]onour, reputation and the stuff of moral careers" remain precious to a person with dementia, as to everyone (Sabat and Harré 1992, 454).

In this chapter I use a case study to explore nuances of the subjective experience of disorientation as expressed in social interaction in the context of dementia care. I focus on residents' personal stakes and concerns about spatiality and place as they simultaneously position themselves in relation to a *moral* landscape.

Moral Landscapes in Positioning Theory

Positioning theory uses spatial metaphors—"positions" as features of a "moral landscape"—to analytically approach aspects of meaning-making having to do with the normative frames people live by (Harré 2010). This involves how people assume and ascribe to each other rights and duties and how actions are taken up as social acts in the interaction. Positions are defined as the "clusters of moral (normative) presuppositions that people believe or are told or slip into and to which they are momentarily bound in what they say and do" (Harré 2010, 53).

Positions are not fixed, but dependent on the subtle shifts of perspectives that evolve in the unfolding interaction—implicitly in how the participants act and more or less explicitly in their conversation. Any positioning act can be challenged in the interaction; in that sense positioning has a power dimension. It is also a matter of being able to present oneself as a "good" and responsible person. Each position entails its own logic through which actions make sense and are morally motivated and justified. People draw on public discourses to position themselves and others in the ongoing conversation. Through the process of mutual positioning, a person's self is discursively constructed (Davies and Harré 1990).

People with dementia continue, even at stages with disorientation problems, to position themselves in relation to whatever rights and duties they perceive as relevant, and with respect to moral projects brought about in the storylines through which they make sense of their lives. However, in doing so, their agency is fragile—not only because of the disease itself, but also because of the social dynamics through which positions are recognized as relevant, made available, and taken up in the interaction.

I refer to agency here as the ability to actively take part in the positioning process instead of just being passively positioned by others. I do not intend to address issues of moral accountability, ethical dilemmas, or any ethical theory. Rather, in dialogue with the data and in line with Davies and Harré (1990) and Harré (2010), I take an interest in positioning as something that is embedded in social life and that is always more or less morally charged from the perspectives of the persons involved.

Care Settings as Venues for Social and Moral Action

Keeping in mind the metaphor of moral landscapes, I now invite you to think of positioning as something that takes place morally (normatively) and spatially at the same time. In line with this, Aminzadeh et al. (2009) found that persons with dementia expressed ambivalent sentiments about the residential facility to which they had recently been relocated. It seems that the setting had a moral dimension to these residents, as it had bearing on the normative frames of their everyday lives.

On one hand, the setting was associated with well-deserved rest, hospitality, and freedom from burdensome chores—a place "designed to serve older people who wish to retire from an active and demanding lifestyle" (Aminzadeh et al. 2009, 493). This image helped residents to position themselves as relatively healthy, independent, competent, and self-reliant. On the other hand, they were concerned about how this way of life imposed restrictions on their abilities to make meaningful contributions. The relocation not only required adjustment to new routines, but also demanded the ability to establish new social roles and identities—or, in terms of positioning, to find other discourses and frameworks to draw on in presenting themselves as morally responsible people. The residents were engaged in what Aminzadeh and coworkers describe as a process of life review and self-scrutiny, reminiscing about personality traits, coping styles, and past experiences of overcoming other challenges in life.

Residential care in general sets boundaries on residents' positioning insofar as their everyday actions have to fit into a local framework of institutional order and routines. This framework offers a repertoire of possible action, more or less well-matched to a person's construction of self. However restricted, agency may still be expressed in strategic use of the repertoire that is nevertheless available (Harnett 2010). People with dementia, as the disease progresses, not only have limited influence on their environment, but in suffering from disorientation, they also lose control of the available repertoire for social and moral action, making their acts of positioning even more fragile.

PLACING THE PLACE, AND PLACING ONESELF WITHIN IT

Focusing on place rather than on disorientation as a disease symptom, a number of researchers in the dementia care field argue for the need to reconstruct congruent environments. "Homeliness" should be evident not only on the surface, with architecture and furnishings, but also in daily routines and interaction. Thereby, it is maintained, residents with dementia will have a familiar frame of reference to hold on to. This will enable them to "know" where they are, understand the place, and act in socially meaningful ways. This contrasts with what has been described in terms of "placelessness" (Briller and Calkins 2000), "dissonant" or "incongruent milieus" (Diaz Moore 1999), "displacement" or "dislocation" (Milligan 2003), or being "out of place" (Calkins and Marsden 2000).

Residential care settings will probably always suffer from some degree of incongruity due to their unavoidable ambiguity as both homes and care institutions. Ethnologist Öhlander (1996) describes the frame of homeliness in dementia care as a "benign fabrication." He found that the frame of care was withheld from the residents; the reason for their stay was undercommunicated, which made the setting confusing for them. Features regarding safety and care practice, which might differ from those of a private home, were never explained—let alone the fact that the residents had to share their "home" with others. Furnishings were a mix of personal and institutional articles, but when somebody did interpret the place as her own private home, this caused trouble. Caregivers sometimes had to take measures to restore order and calm, such as by changing the furnishings and décor.

SETTING THE STAGE FOR SOCIAL AND MORAL ACTION

Incongruities of the care environment, as those described above, may cause residents "to be unsure of how to act and what to expect within this setting" (Weber 2000, 24). Öhlander (1996) found that despite all efforts to make residents feel at home in the facility, they often seemed to wonder where they were. Their interpretations of the place were unstable. Applying a variety of familiar frameworks, they would transform the setting into a school, a nursing home, or a dinner party. At meals, the ladies residing in the unit would alternately assume the positions of guests and hostesses.

This is not unique to residential care; similar observations have been reported from day-hospital settings. In one case the occupational activities were perceived as a school where one did as one was told and tried to give proper answers, as a pupil, and took no other initiatives. In contrast, the person's own home afforded an arena for more responsible action and allowed her to position herself, with certain moral stature, as the gracious hostess (Borell et al. 1994). In residential care there may be no such alternative arena for the person, hence the consequences of perceived lack of influence, authority, and rights are greater.

Observational studies illustrate how places are negotiated among residents with dementia at times with little staff involvement. The setting may form the stage for more private talk or territorial claims (Diaz Moore 1999) or transform into something else—such as a private home where "guests" are entertained (Zingmark, Norberg, and Sandman 1993). Some frameworks are more enabling than others. As reported in a previous case study from dementia care (Örulv

2010), one resident's frightening image of the place was met with another resident's more constructive interpretation. Eventually it was co-constructed as a venue for social activity in line with previous experiences and thus rendered socially as well as personally meaningful.

On closer observation even "inaccurate" interpretations may not only follow a rather plausible logic, but also fill a moral and social void. It has been suggested elsewhere that they provide guidelines for how to act and allow the persons to make claims about themselves as driven by certain values (Örulv and Hydén 2006). However vulnerable to difficulties in the interaction, such attempts to make sense of the situation show the potential and need for meaning-driven and agentive action among people with dementia.

The Case of Sunny Glade

In a six-month ethnographic research project, I made video-recordings at a Swedish elder center, referred to here as "Sunny Glade," focusing on a dementia unit with eight residents (see Örulv 2008). As I was intrigued by the dramas that took place from the perspectives of the residents, data were collected in an "improvising" mode. In deciding what to record I was sensitive to the action and drama I was able to perceive at the time. One such episode of "drama" forms the basis for this chapter. The episode illustrates how their vague understanding of the place gives two female residents trouble in their daily life—they do not know how to behave and where to go, or whether to stay or leave. For them the displayed disorientation takes the shape of a *moral* problem, or a matter of what is socially expected from a decent person, rather than an issue of way-finding or memory. The participants are relatively articulate about their concerns in conversation, which makes them accessible for analysis. The varying degrees to which an assistant nurse is involved in the communication add to the complexity of the episode.

The main characters of the drama are Martha and Catherine, diagnosed with Alzheimer's disease 4–5 and 7–8 years ago, respectively, who have developed a close friendship here. Both in their nineties, they are still quite physically fit and often engage in conversation with each other. Martha is more inclined to hold the floor and generally less linguistically impaired (see Hydén and Örulv 2009). Catherine has some trouble recognizing objects in her surroundings. Both women have severe memory problems and often display disorientation in place and time.

The chosen episode involves Martha and Catherine spending some time in the local dayroom just before afternoon coffee. For staff, it is the time of the day when one shift ends and another begins. Assistant nurse Eve, seated next to the ladies, has to attend to some administrative tasks—writing reports and giving her coworker Joseph the day's debriefing as he arrives for the evening shift. Occasionally she leaves the room for errands or chores.

PROLOGUE: HAPPENINGS CONTRIBUTING TO DISORIENTATION

Prior to this scene Martha and Catherine have accompanied assistant nurse Anita, from the day shift, on the nurse's errand of borrowing a book for later reading-aloud sessions. As the three of them come back to the unit, Martha and Catherine seem to be at a loss what to do while Anita gets busy sorting out some practical matter with a colleague in the kitchen. After a while, they sit down at one of the kitchen tables but remain attentive to what Anita is doing. From what can be heard from their conversation, it seems that Martha searches the environment for clues of where they are. She recognizes some of the décor and suggests that they may actually have come back to where they live.

Still, when Anita is about to leave the kitchen, Catherine alerts Martha, and they immediately tag along. Anita assembles a group of armchairs in the day room to get started with the book before it is time for her to leave her shift, but it turns out that Catherine needs to use the toilet and Anita escorts her to her private room. In the meantime I start to set up the recording equipment in the day room. After a while Martha very politely asks me if she could use the ladies' room too, and I tell her "But of course!" Martha explains that they are in the company of the woman "who lives here" (to which I, taken aback, reply "Oh, I see"). Then she hurries away to Catherine's room. Anita stops her and shows her to her own room instead. Now there won't be any time for reading or following up on their errand by talking about the book.

"AREN'T YOU GOING HOME TODAY THEN?"

When the ladies show up in the day room again, it is time for Anita and another colleague to leave. As they explain this and say their goodbyes, Catherine remarks with surprise (and perhaps some annoyance) "What, are we to leave *again*?" The distress of another resident, pleading for Anita to stay, demands full attention from staff. Therefore little notice is taken of Martha and Catherine in their confusion. Martha turns to Catherine and asks her,

Excerpt 1

Martha: But…but *listen*, aren't you going home today then?
Catherine: Well I suppose I have to.

Eve:	Nooo. You *live* here in (name of neighborhood).
Catherine:	Oh?
Eve:	You are at Sunny Glade now.
Martha:	Yes at Sunny Glade yes.
Eve:	Yes, X Street five. In (name of neighborhood).
Catherine:	Where is that?
Eve:	*X Street* is where it is.
Catherine:	X Street (Eve: Uh-huh) *five.*
Eve:	Uh-huh. Sunny Glade.
Martha:	Sunny Glade precisely yes. (whispers)
Eve:	You have … your own apartments. Where you went to the toilet just now.
Martha:	Nooo (in a sceptical tone of voice) but *I* I uh I *was* at Sunny Glade now, wasn't I?
Eve:	Uh-huh?
Martha:	Yes. But that's not in the same place as
Eve:	Yes, you live in the same place.
Martha:	Is it?
Eve:	Yes. You but you have your room closer here (makes gestures) and Catherine has hers a bit further down.
Martha:	I see.
Eve:	In the hallway.
Martha:	Yes. That's how it is. (low voice)
Eve:	Further down the hallway, uh-huh.
Catherine:	Uh-huh. (bends forward to look at the borrowed book in front of her)
Eve:	Have you been borrowing some books? I saw.
Catherine:	*Nooo.* We haven't.
Eve:	Oh but didn't you go with Anita to borrow some books?
Martha:	"Mia … at … Brunnskull-" (book title) nooo. (low voice that turns to a whisper; pauses) Isn't that it? (whispers) (pause)
Eve:	Weren't you down at Sophie's (the nurse) to borr look at some books? (pause)
Catherine:	No?
Eve:	Just now? Hnn?
Catherine:	No?

People with dementia in residential care are often found to be "homesick" or trying to find their way to a home that existed in the past. Several authors have described this "displaced" quest for home as a search for sanctuary, security, and emotional shelter when the world around them is confusing (e.g., Bowlby Sifton 2000; Zingmark, Norberg and Sandman 1993). Interestingly, in this episode Martha and Catherine do not seem that eager to go home. The way they talk about it, going home could very well be something they feel *obligated* to do; after all, others are heading home and it may seem like the decent thing to do. As the assistant nurse explains that Martha and Catherine live there at Sunny Glade, in their own private rooms, they seem content with that. They immediately drop the subject of going home and instead request further details about their current address, repeating the information as if to imprint it into their memory. Yet some confusion remains, which is further illustrated as the episode unfolds.

Some of this case's confusion could most likely be attributed to the fact that Martha and Catherine have just returned from the nurse's office, in another part of the building, passing through other corridors and day rooms quite similar to their own. I cannot tell from the video data whether Anita emphasizes the fact that they have now come back to where they started. Apparently this is not so obvious for the ladies. That could be what Martha is referring to as she suggests that she *was* at Sunny Glade and this is not the same place. Perhaps that is what Eve realizes, too, as she asks about it. By now Catherine seems to have forgotten about their errand, though, or perhaps her interpretation of it did not involve specifically going to the nurse's or borrowing a book. Eve's attempt to orient the ladies to place and situation is hampered by difficulties in finding a common frame of reference in the communication.

What strikes me in this sequence is how the participants shift between different modes when talking about place and spatiality. Catherine's spontaneous remark—"What, are we to leave *again*?"—refers to the fact that they have recently moved from one location to another. At the same time it alludes to some kind of expectation, as in being (potentially) expected to leave. The tone of surprise in her voice indicates that she, herself, had expected that they would stay at least for a while after their arrival/return. This constitutes a social mode, involving repertoires for how spatial matters (leaving, staying) are usually handled. Martha brings up the idea of going home, which is taken as something one *has* to do—a moral mode is being invoked, referring to duty. The different modes are also reflected in Eve's attempts to explain to the ladies where they are. She invokes their status as residents living there and having their own apartments (moral mode, implying rights), refers to social meanings of the place (name of the facility and neighborhood, their borrowing books at the nurses' office), as well as provides an explanation of where their rooms are located (way-finding). This short sequence illustrates the complexity of our spatial relations, the coherence of which we normally just take for granted without further reflection.

At this time the conversation is interrupted by Joseph coming from the changing room and asking what is up today. Then, both assistant nurses talk about the influenza currently affecting the unit.

MORAL AGENTS, MORAL ARENAS

As Joseph leaves for the kitchen, Eve turns to the ladies to make conversation, asking whether they feel like having coffee (something of a cultural institution in Sweden). The ensuing conversation reveals some uncertainty of what would be the appropriate action. First Catherine spontaneously acknowledges that she does, soon, whereas her friend Martha says in a low voice "No, we don't." Catherine then immediately makes a gesture indicating embarrassment, as if she has committed a faux pas. She raises her shoulders and bends over, covering her face with her hand, then looks up and smiles apologetically. Stuttering, "No it's not it's not," she turns her gaze to Eve, who intervenes:

Excerpt 2

Eve:	It is time for coffee soon. So it's about time for you to want coffee. Then it is about time soon. (smiles and nods throughout the utterance)
Martha:	But that's we'll have that at Sunny Glade then, I suppose?
Eve:	Yes, 'll serve it here (points to the group of sofa and arm chairs next to them) (?: uh-huh) precisely.
Martha:	Oh I see?
Eve:	Uh-huh.
?:	Yes. Well thank you!
Eve:	This is Sunny Glade now.
Martha:	Yes we are at Sunny Glade now.
Eve:	Yes we are there now.
Catherine:	I don't know if I brought any money with me?
Eve:	But that's already paid for, it's included in your rent.
Catherine:	Oh!
Eve:	In the rent that you pay for your room all food and snacks are included.
Martha:	Yes, that's how it is now. (Catherine nods)
Eve:	Yes, (?: yes) that's good.
Martha:	Yes that's very good indeed.
Eve:	Uh-huh.

Martha's question in the beginning of the excerpt—"But that's we'll have that at Sunny Glade then, I suppose?"—points to some kind of problem. It could be interpreted as something between an objection (but not *here*?!), a suggestion (to have coffee at Sunny Glade as usual), and a request for clarification (we *are* having coffee at *Sunny Glade*, aren't we?). Presumably Martha does not recognize being back at Sunny Glade (or the part of Sunny Glade that she knows by that name). To Martha, being at Sunny Glade seems to provide a framework allowing her to enjoy her coffee as usual—as long as she recognizes that she is in fact there. Catherine, on the other hand, expresses concerns about being able to pay. The name Sunny Glade does not seem to have the same familiar ring to her, with social connotations and a normative framework, as to Martha. With Eve's place orientation and explanations that coffee is included in the rent and already paid for, both ladies seem relieved and content.

However, as Eve somewhat later (in talking to another resident) says that she will prepare some coffee, Martha seems to have forgotten about the earlier information. Seemingly uncomfortable, she says in a low voice, "Oh, but you shouldn't." This time Eve does not explain where they are or that coffee is included. Instead she invokes a less formal framework:

Excerpt 3

Eve:	Coffee and ca– but certainly we must have coffee and cake?!
Catherine:	Certainly we must have coffee.
Eve:	Yes, certainly one must. (laughs)
Catherine:	Otherwise one might *pass away* at an early age. (puts her hand to her heart in a theatrical gesture)
Eve:	(laughs) Yes, that's never any good.
Catherine:	Noo! (austere tone of voice, smiling slyly)
Martha:	We should invite her over some afternoon as well.
Eve:	(giggles)
Catherine:	Yes.
Martha:	Certainly.
Eve:	(giggles) Uh-huh.
Martha:	Why not?
Eve:	Well, you're doing fine.

One could perhaps say that Eve in Excerpt 3 above appeals to a discourse of allowing oneself to indulge in the good things of life occasionally—a discourse that is compatible with the image of a place for well-deserved hospitality and rest. In doing so, she does not position herself as a caregiver providing services, however, but more as a fellow human being sharing the same need for an afternoon treat. This strategy is well received by Catherine. It allows her to engage in a dialogue full of wit in what seems to be a socially rewarding framework for her. Catherine and Eve are elegantly attuned to each other in the interaction, filling in on each other's sentences in the same jocular manner as a team. Catherine mimics Eve's shifting tempo and her tone of voice, and Eve plays along with Catherine's suggestion that refraining from having coffee could actually be fatal. Attentive interaction with staff being fully present with the residents, valuing them as persons and striving for some common ground, has been found to promote a sense of at-homeness (ease, expressions of content, or joy) in dementia care (Eggers, Norberg, and Ekman 2005; Edvardsson, Sandman, and Rasmussen 2011; Zingmark, Norberg, and Sandman 1993). In this case, Catherine seems to feel at home in the situation and no longer shows any signs of embarrassment.

However, this discourse leaves Martha's uncertainty and moral concerns unresolved. As argued by Aminzadeh et al. (2009), while allowing for greater comfort and freedom from an earlier, more demanding lifestyle, the notion of hospitality and rest also involves an erosion of agency. Instead of doing things for others, residents must now adjust to having things done for *them*. This does not come very easily to Martha, who takes great pride both in her independence and in her history of being generous and helpful to others, as is evident in her many stories (see Hydén and Örulv 2009; Örulv and Hydén 2006).

It should be noted that in this sequence Martha is left with the belief that she and her friend are being treated to coffee by this young woman, Eve. This makes Martha uncomfortable enough not only to insist on inviting her back some other time, as was shown in Excerpt 3; as the episode unfolds, she also argues for a change of arena. When Eve temporarily leaves the room to get a report book from the kitchen, Martha turns to Catherine to suggest that they all go to Sunny Glade for coffee instead. Eve returns just in time to establish, once again, that they are in fact at Sunny Glade. This is met with surprise and, on Martha's part, with lingering uncertainty ("But I have been to Sunny Glade now so I so I guess I'm still *there* then, I guess I'm still *there* then...I don't know."). The topic of having coffee at Sunny Glade (instead) is brought up again a couple of times; Sunny Glade is depicted as a place where coffee is included in Martha's rent. Finally Martha approaches Eve directly to suggest that she join them for coffee at Sunny Glade. Not quite apprehending the generous offer, Eve assures Martha that she will have some coffee too.

The examples above illustrate difficulties that may arise in the mutual positioning within the care setting. They point to a perceived lack of ability to take (moral) action. The fact that Martha is so concerned about shifting to another arena (where she in fact happens to be already, albeit unknowingly) indicates this matter's importance to her. Presumably she perceives that her current situation and location do not satisfactorily support her positioning herself as a morally responsible person. From her point of view, by moving to a more suitable arena she would be able to claim a certain moral stature as the generous hostess or at least as someone who is paying her way. Martha wants to go someplace where she is (morally) in control of the situation.

Within the logic of care practice, Martha's concerns are somewhat misdirected. Not only does she fail to recognize that she and the others are already (or still) at Sunny Glade, but also her frame of reference does not apply to the way coffee is handled in the unit. Within the discourse of care, there is no need for residents to be concerned about generosity and reciprocity. Although acknowledging the ladies' polite offering earlier of having her over for coffee some time, Eve does not really express any gratitude. She does not assume the position as someone for whom that would be relevant. From her point of view, coffee time is nothing but a nice daily routine and a task to be accomplished for the residents' benefit—nowhere near the drama apparently taking place from Martha's perspective where places are so elusive and yet so morally relevant.

Another way of putting this would be that the discursive practices of residential care fail to take into account the logic in which Martha positions herself as a moral agent. Thus, in the interaction she is unable to make determinate those actions that could fulfill the normative expectations incorporated by her position (cf. Davies and Harré 1990). In that sense she is, in her own logic, robbed of agency—at least as long as there is no other way for her to live up to her values.

JUSTIFYING PRESENCE

The difficulties in relating to the place on a moral level are further demonstrated in Excerpt 4 below, in which Eve has left the room to prepare for coffee and collect the other residents. In the excerpt it is clear that Martha and Catherine do not readily recognize the dayroom as theirs to lay claim to, as is intended. Left alone in the room, they discuss whether or not they are in the right place and whether their timing is right. While Catherine mainly expresses feelings of being abandoned, Martha seems even more concerned about her right to stay in this place. In their discussion Martha refers to a conversation with some local authority figure, invoking her rightful claim to the place based on the erroneous premise that her (late) husband is working there. Seemingly she feels a need to legitimize her presence. However shaky the grounds invoked, and however hesitantly, Martha is able to verbally position herself as someone who is not trespassing on somebody else's territory. By her own account, she has properly announced their visit in advance. Even if they have been forgotten, they were supposed to be there today.

Excerpt 4

Catherine:	We weren't all that important. (looks around, then makes eye contact with Martha)
Martha:	Huh?
Catherine:	I guess we weren't all that important. Why, they were to come here to talk to us (looks around) but (inaudible) *up* (waves her hand in the air), just.
Martha:	Yes.
Catherine:	So where did they go?
Martha:	Yes they did, but we're staying here anyway, aren't we.
Catherine:	(makes a smacking sound, looks down briefly, then up)
Martha:	But they said... 'cause I guess they weren't sure. But then I told them that I'm... well... (husband's name) he works has his work here and
Catherine:	I see.
Martha:	I said. And uh... and they know that I'll be here I said.
Catherine:	Uh-*huh* (nods).
Martha:	Because so I've... told them. That we were coming,
Catherine:	I see.
Martha:	and (husband's name) said so too that we were com– Yes well they didn't bother. To listen to us.
Catherine:	I see.
Martha:	(It) was so certain so certain then. (tone of indignation or bitter sarcasm)
Catherine:	I see. So she didn't say any certain... *name* then? Of the day?
Martha:	Huh?
Catherine:	They didn't say any certain name of the day? (pause) What day we eh were supposed to be here?
Martha:	Well I suppose that's today.
Catherine:	I see. (low voice)
Martha:	Uh I was *supposed* to come here today.
Catherine:	Oh. (low voice)

Then Eve arrives with the other residents, announcing in a singsong voice that they are all welcome to coffee. Spirits are high as Eve shows the residents to their seats. Eve puts her arm around Martha, who now has a big smile on her face, and shouts with laughter as Martha (literally) tickles her ribs. Catherine is humming happily.

Earlier research has found that even short moments without a caregiver present in the room may result in feelings of abandonment and patients being "on their way home" (Zingmark, Norberg, and Sandman 1993). This kind of anxiety is likely to emanate, to a great extent, from a decreasing amount of attentive interaction and, as a consequence, from feelings of being unrelated (not at home) in the present (Eggers, Norberg, and Ekman 2005; Zingmark, Norberg, and Sandman 1993). The emotional tone differs significantly depending on whether staff members have to focus on tasks and routines or have the time to interact and be fully present with the residents (Edvardsson, Sandman, and Rasmussen 2011). Undoubtedly, this has strong relevance for the anxiety displayed in Excerpt 4.

Still, I contend that the unclear social and moral expectations of the dementia care setting also play a predominant part—perhaps *especially* at times of less staff involvement, when there is little social guidance available. The anxiety, the uncertainty, and the need to justify and legitimize one's presence in what is actually supposed to be one's home point to a fundamental problem. Without some grasp of the meaning of the place, what one is doing there, and what kind of relationship one has to the place, one will always be a stranger to it. Thus, however pleasant the place may be, one will never take liberties with it as one would "at home." One will always regard oneself as being at somebody else's mercy, or owing a debt of gratitude to somebody. When left to one's own devices, if only for a few minutes, one will feel abandoned in a way that one would not in familiar territory.

Discussion

Symptoms like disorientation are *lived*; depending on individual life history and patterns for coping, they have different personal significance and are differently dealt with. How they take shape is also highly dependent on environmental context—clues in the setting (as associated with known frameworks), conversational cues, and the familiar discourses that are introduced. The examples in this explorative case study illustrate what a profound impact deeply rooted values may have in the nuances of everyday life, in spite of rather severe memory and orientation problems. We could see that everyday happenings, such as staff changing shift and the prospect of having coffee, may raise an abundance of moral concerns with respect to spatiality in a broad sense. Matters of staying, leaving, returning, going somewhere, and recognizing a place, are intertwined not only with frameworks of what is socially meaningful, but also with *moral* frameworks of how things should be done.

Being on one's way somewhere, in a disoriented manner, may be an attempt to seek out an arena offering better opportunity for moral action and for claiming the position of a morally responsible person. This could be, for instance, as a proud woman paying her way rather than relying on the mercy and generosity of others and burdening other people. Similarly, residents may feel the need to justify and legitimize their presence in the residential facility, as if they had no right to feel at home there. Referring to a legitimate reason for being there and to arrangements with persons that one believes have righteous claims to the place, however inaccurately, could be a strategy for claiming moral agency.

In the entire corpus of data, this kind of anxiety is recurring. There are instances where residents are not sure whether or not they are expected or allowed to stay—at the dining-table if one has already eaten, or in the setting as a whole when not paid attention to by staff. They often express concerns about how to pay for coffee, meals, or lodging, or show embarrassment because they perceive themselves as dependent on others' generosity. One resident is sometimes distressed because she believes that she is paying for everyone else as well, which she sees as a violation of her rights. Residents also express uncertainty of their responsibilities within the setting, or assume responsibilities on false grounds, both of which can be very stressful. In times of little staff involvement, a relatively less impaired resident often perceives that the responsibility for taking care of others is hers. She may even, hence, refrain from leaving until the more impaired person appears to manage by himself or herself, as if it were her duty to stay with him or her. Unclear expectations may thus have direct bearing on spatial behavior and cause much unnecessary anxiety—apart from the cognitive exhaustion I imagine would be the result of such constant interpretive work, *especially* with cognitive dysfunction.

It has been argued before that in order for residents to feel at home, careful consideration of person-environment congruence is required. This includes personal meanings of home and personal values, fears, desire, and expectations, and in a continuous process of adjustment (Aminzadeh et al. 2009). My argument is that persons with dementia need to be taken seriously as moral agents in the sense that they strive to lead a good life according to their values. Care practice thus needs to be more sensitive to their moral concerns and stakes in daily life.

With a systematic team effort, caregivers could map out what situations might involve moral stakes and concerns for each unique individual residing in the facility, with respect to life history and values. This could be done as part of an ongoing life-review process. The next step would be to consider what would relieve each of them of their distress. Discourses and frameworks need to be flexible enough to address a variety of concerns and stakes without apparent conflicts. For instance, allowing oneself a treat in the afternoon, in convivial company, *need not* be in conflict with knowing that one has paid for it properly already.

Much could be gained from making residents less dependent on constant orientation and reminders from staff. Visible cues could guide residents not only to where they are, but also to what they are welcome to do, what services are available free of charge, and so on. Such relatively simple measures could be helpful in providing frameworks and repertoires for action.

This alone would not entirely solve the need to fulfill moral values that have been the guiding stars throughout one's life—now threatened both by decreasing abilities and by institutional practice restrictions. It remains essential to provide opportunities for residents to contribute in meaningful ways on their own terms and, successively, to help them let go of responsibilities. Such issues are the fundaments of serious life crises that might require substantial psychological support, something that is rarely available in dementia care today. As we learn more about the subjective experiences of people with dementia and take their personal stakes and concerns seriously, we may need to find ways to address this lack of support.

References

Aminzadeh, Faranak, William B. Dalziel, Frank J. Molnar, and Linda J. Garcia. 2009. "Symbolic Meaning of Relocation to a Residential Care Facility for Persons with Dementia." *Aging & Mental Health* 13 (3): 487–496.

Borell, Lena, Anders Gustavsson, Per-Olof Sandman, and Gary Kielhofner. 1994. "Occupational Programming in a Day Hospital for Patients with Dementia." *The Occupational Therapy Journal of Research* 14 (4): 219–238.

Bowlby Sifton, Carol. 2000. "Searching for Home." *Alzheimer's Care Quarterly* 1 (1): 8–16.

Briller, Sherylyn, and Margaret P. Calkins. 2000. "Defining Place-based Models of Care: Conceptualizing Care Settings as Home, Resort, or Hospital." *Alzheimer's Care Quarterly* 1 (1): 17–23.

Calkins, Margaret P., and John P. Marsden. 2000. "Home is Where the Heart Is: Designing to Recreate Home." *Alzheimer's Care Quarterly* 1 (1): 8–16.

Davies, Bronwyn, and Rom Harré. 1990. "Positioning: The Discursive Production of Selves." *Journal for the Theory of Social Behaviour* 20 (1): 43–63.

Diaz Moore, Keith. 1999. "Dissonance in the Dining Room: A Study of Social Interaction in a Special Care Unit." *Qualitative Health Research* 9 (1): 133–155.

Edvardsson, David, Per-Olof Sandman, and Birgit Rasmussen. 2011. "Forecasting the Ward Climate: A Study from a Dementia Care Unit." *Journal of Clinical Nursing* 21: 1136–1144.

Eggers, Thomas, Astrid Norberg, and Sirkka-Liisa Ekman. 2005. "Counteracting Fragmentation in the Care of People with Moderate and Severe Dementia." *Clinical Nursing Research* 14 (4): 343–369.

Harnett, Tove. 2010. "Seeking Exemption from Nursing Home Routines: Residents' Everyday Influence Attempts and Institutional Order." *Journal of Aging Studies* 24: 292–301.

Harré, Rom. 2010. "Positioning as a Metagrammar for Discursive Story Lines." In *Telling Stories: Language, Narrative, and Social Life*, edited by Deborah Schiffrin, Anna De Fina, and Anastasia Nylund. Washington: Georgetown University Press, Georgetown University Round Table on Languages and Linguistics Series.

Hydén, Lars-Christer, and Linda Örulv. 2009. "Narrative and Identity in Alzheimer's Disease: A Case Study." *Journal of Ageing Studies* 23: 205–214.

Milligan, Christine. 2003. "Location or Dis-location? Towards a Conceptualization of People and Place in the Care-giving Experience." *Social & Cultural Geography* 4 (4): 455–470.

Öhlander, Magnus. 1996. "Skör verklighet. En Etnologisk Studie av Demensvård i Gruppboende." [A Fragile Reality. An Ethnological Study of Dementia Care in Group Dwelling.] PhD diss., Institutet för Folklivsforskning, Stockholm University, Sweden.

Örulv, Linda. 2008. "Fragile Identities, Patched-up Worlds. Dementia and Meaning-making in Social Interaction." PhD diss., Department of Medical and Health Sciences, Division of Health and Society, Linköping University, Sweden. Available electronically at Linköping University Electronic press: http://liu.diva-portal.org/smash/record.jsf?pid=diva2:18145&rvn=2.

Örulv, Linda. 2010. "Placing the Place, and Placing Oneself Within it: (Dis)orientation and (Dis)continuity in Dementia." *Dementia: The International Journal of Social Research and Practice* 9 (1): 21–44.

Örulv, Linda, and Lars-Christer Hydén. 2006. "Confabulation: Sense-making, Self-making and World-making in Dementia." *Discourse Studies* 8 (5): 647–673.

Sabat, Steven R., and Rom Harré. 1992. "The Construction and Deconstruction of Self in Alzheimer's Disease." *Ageing and Society* 12: 443–461.

Vittoria, Anne K. 1999. "'Our Own Little Language': Naming and the Social Construction of Alzheimer's Disease." *Symbolic Interaction* 22 (4): 361–384.

Weber, Chari. 2000. "A Place Story of Home: Using Stories to Enhance Facility Comprehension and Integration of Place-based Models of Care." *Alzheimer's Care Quarterly* 1 (1): 24–34.

Westius, Anders, Lars Andersson, and Kjell Kallenberg. 2009. "View of Life in Persons with Dementia." *Dementia: The International Journal of Social Research and Practice* 8 (4): 481–499.

Westius, Anders, Kjell Kallenberg, and Astrid Norberg. 2010. "Views of Life and Sense of Identity in People with Alzheimer's Disease." *Ageing and Society* 30 (7): 1257–1278.

Zingmark, Karin, Astrid Norberg, and Per-Olof Sandman. 1993. "Experience of At-homeness and Homesickness in Patients with Alzheimer's Disease." *The American Journal of Alzheimer's Care and Related Disorders & Research* 8: 10–16.

Index

acquired brain injury, 4, 91–95, 104–105
agency, 2–3, 5, 7, 12, 21, 73, 95–96, 109–112, 192–193, 201, 202, 205
Alive Inside, 107, 116
Alzheimer's disease, 2, 5, 12, 18–19, 21–22, 24, 28, 53, 55–56, 59–60, 70, 92–93, 98, 102, 108–112, 114, 123, 137, 191, 195
Aristotle, 12–15, 50, 111
autobiographical, 4, 70, 72, 74–76, 78, 80, 82–87, 140
autobiographical time, 70, 74, 84
autonomy, 43–45, 48, 51, 54, 56, 64, 102
autotelic goals, 30–32, 34–35

basic intentionality, 112–113
Basting, Anne, 54–55, 86, 103
being-in-the-world, 113, 123
bio-psycho-social model of dementia, 24–25
biographical, 64, 70, 72, 177–178, 180–181, 187
biography, 173, 176, 179, 182–183, 185–186
bodily schema, 113–114
body, 4–5, 17, 19, 27–28, 46, 49, 51, 54, 72, 93, 109–117, 120–123, 128–129, 131–133
  selfhood, 4–5, 109–117
  lived, 5, 49, 112, 121–122
Bourdieu, Pierre, 5, 112–113, 115–116
brain, 4, 12, 27–28, 69, 72–75, 80–84, 91, 92–98, 101–105, 110–111, 116–117, 120, 122, 142
  injury, 4, 27, 73, 91–98, 101–105
Bratman, Michael, 20, 141, 143, 145
Bruner, Jerome, 76, 141, 147, 148
Bullington, Jennifer, 49

Calnan, Michael, 46
caregiver, 3, 6, 19, 35, 64–66, 191, 194, 200, 203, 205
  family, 3, 25, 55, 97, 101, 146, 155
  formal, 25, 62, 64, 156, 169, 186
case study, 7, 192, 194, 204

Cavell, Stanley, 15–16
child, 15, 16, 18, 19, 20, 42, 50, 61–63, 71, 100, 102–103, 120, 125, 131, 137, 141, 147–148
  adult, 1, 55, 61–63, 100, 102–103
  childhood, 13, 55, 60, 63, 116, 127, 130
Clark, Andy, 73
Clark, Herbert, 141, 144–145
Clegg, David, 85–86
collaboration, 1, 6–7, 139–143, 146, 148, 152
comparative analysis, 4, 92, 104–105
comprehension, 155–156, 158–161, 163–170
conarration, 95–97
continuity, sense of sameness, 4, 75, 85, 87, 117, 129
conversation, 2, 6, 7, 28, 29, 31–32, 71, 97, 101–103, 108, 124, 137–138, 141–143, 146–148, 150, 169, 170, 181, 192, 195–196, 199, 202
  analysis, 155, 171
  interaction, 141–142, 146, 148, 150, 155, 157–161, 163–165
  storytelling, 7, 97, 101–103, 138, 147, 181, 192
corporeality, 110–111, 117
couplehood, 53, 56, 63–65, 143
creativity, 86, 116, 177
critical personalism, 2, 24, 26–27
culture, 35, 50, 55, 72, 81, 115, 178

day care centre, 6, 27, 56, 96, 155–156, 162, 166, 169–171
dementia, 1–7, 12, 18, 34, 35, 39, 46–51, 53–61, 64–65, 69–71, 73, 75–77, 80, 83–86, 92–98, 100–105, 107, 109–113, 115, 117, 120–125, 127, 129, 131–133, 139, 144, 149, 150–151, 155–156, 158, 160, 163, 165–166, 169–170, 173–181, 183–187, 191–195, 197, 201, 205–206

209

dementia (*Cont.*)
  advanced, 127, 144, 149
  diagnosed with, 6, 24, 25, 27, 29, 31, 34, 35, 55, 56, 61, 71, 78, 80, 91, 174, 195
  early/young onset, 5, 6, 93, 94, 173–183
  experience of, 5–7, 25, 27, 31, 35, 48, 49, 55, 71, 85–86, 93, 121–125, 174–176, 178–179, 183–185, 206
  living with, 3, 5, 24, 53–56, 64, 71, 86, 121–122, 173, 176, 178, 183, 185
Dewey, John, 110, 123–124
dignified, 40–41, 46, 51
Dignitas, 40
dignity, 2–3, 34, 39–51, 53–54, 56, 62–64
discourse, socio-cultural, 40, 46, 54, 63, 72, 76–78, 80, 109–110, 112, 121–122, 192–193, 200–202, 204, 205
  in talk, 96, 99, 101–102, 184
Drew, Paul, 157, 166
dualism, 117, 122–123

Edgar, Andrew, 39, 43
embodied, 4–5, 14, 75, 77, 85, 113–117, 122–123, 125, 127–128, 130, 132–133
  meaning, 5, 115, 132
  selfhood, 5, 109, 111–113, 117
emotion, 5, 17, 24, 28, 34, 48–51, 81, 94–95, 110, 132, 198, 204
existential, 73, 94, 109, 112, 113, 114
experience, temporal, 74–75, 81–83, 85
  lived, 91, 120–122, 184–185

face-saving, 101–102
family, 2, 30, 59–60, 76, 92, 94, 96–104, 124, 126–127
  caregiving, 3–7, 25, 155, 173–187
  interaction, 2, 5, 7, 92, 97, 101–102, 104
Franklin, Lise-Lotte, 48
Freeman, Mark, 86–87

Goldstein, Kurt, 73, 95
Goodwin, Charles, 141–142
Gopnik, Alison, 20

habitus, 112–113, 115–116
Hauser, Kaspar, 19–21
Heidegger, Martin, 123, 132
Herzog, Werner, 19
heterotelic goals, 30–35
hope, 11, 85, 94–95, 103
human rights, 44–45

imagination, 81, 83, 86
identity, 1–5, 7, 17, 18, 40, 42–49, 54–56, 64, 69–72, 74–80, 83–87, 93–97, 102, 104, 121–122, 129, 131–132

autobiographical, 4, 70, 74–76, 82–87
intersubjective, 43, 75, 85
integrity, 43, 45, 48, 54, 56, 58
intentionality, 73, 110, 112–115, 117
interaction, conversation, 141–142, 146, 148, 150, 155, 157–161, 163–165
  social, 2, 5–7, 24, 32, 65, 75, 77, 85–86, 92, 96, 97, 101–102, 104, 139–142, 144–152, 155–158, 160, 163, 165–167, 170, 192–193, 195, 201, 202, 204
  problems, 139–140, 142, 144–151, 157–158, 160, 163, 165, 170
interpretation, 4, 25, 81, 95, 99, 102, 123, 144, 157, 164, 183, 194–195, 198

joint activity, 20, 137–139, 141–146, 148–152
joint attention, 144, 170

Kant, Immanuel, 14, 22
Kitwood, Tom, 31, 35, 85, 111, 121–122, 141, 184
Kolnai, Aurel, 43, 51

life story, 26, 56, 58, 60, 63–64, 176
Locke, John, 70, 75, 80, 85, 87, 95, 121
loss of self, 3, 12, 94–95, 109, 121, 176.
  See also: memory
Luria, Alexander, 73

malignant social psychology, 35
Matthews, Eric, 49, 51, 75, 112
McDowell, John, 12, 14–16
meaning, embodied, 5
meaning construction, 4, 6, 82, 145, 148
meaning-making, 4, 82, 92, 148, 192
memory, 4, 69–87, 94, 116, 120–121, 137, 162, 198
  as an archive, 74, 78, 80, 85
  disorder, 70, 72, 86
  loss, 3, 47–48
  problems with, 56–59, 61, 71, 95, 97, 98–100, 103, 108, 195, 204
Menschenwürde, 3, 39, 40, 44–47
Merleau-Ponty, Maurice, 5, 49, 51, 112–115, 117, 123
Mirandola, Pico della, 45
Murdoch, Iris, 53, 55, 65, 70, 71
music, 5, 19, 107–120, 124, 127–133
mutual, 6, 20, 55, 64, 79, 86, 139, 145, 148, 151, 161, 170, 177, 191–192, 201
  positioning, 192, 201
  support, 139, 145, 145, 177
  understanding, 6, 151, 170, 191

narrative, 4, 6, 42, 64, 69, 73, 75–77, 85–86, 94, 95, 97, 99–104, 140, 173–176, 180, 183–185, 187

activity, 17–18, 85, 92
counter, 97, 99, 102, 104
identity, 17–18, 75, 77, 85–86, 95–97, 102, 104
neurodegeneration, 4, 84–85, 93
news receipt tokens, 158, 166–169

person with dementia, 1–3, 7, 24, 34, 39, 46–48, 51, 64, 85–86, 92, 95, 97, 102–104, 112, 122, 139, 144, 149, 151, 155–156, 158, 160, 163, 165, 169, 170, 174–175, 177, 178, 180–181, 184–186, 191, 193, 205
person, status, 12, 18–19, 42, 44, 46–47
responsibility, 73, 96, 101, 139, 147–148, 177, 191–194, 202, 204–206
Person-World Relations, 27, 29
personhood, 2, 3–5,7, 12, 16–22, 70, 74, 77, 85, 95–96, 104, 121–122
phenomenology, 4–5, 85, 124
positioning, 6, 65, 96, 192–193, 201
postautobiographical, 69–70, 83
pre-reflective, 110–117
preservative love, 12, 19, 22
primordial, 5, 111–115, 117

repair, conversational, 6, 143–145, 149–151, 156–158, 161, 163, 166–168
respect, 21–22, 40, 41–45, 47, 54, 71, 73
responses, interactional, 17–19, 101, 109, 140, 144, 146, 149–150, 159, 160–162, 164–165, 169, 178

Rossato-Bennett, Michael, 107
Rousseau, Jean-Jacques, 12–14
Ruddick, Sara, 12, 19

Sacks, Oliver, 116–117
scaffolding, 6, 95, 146–152
Schegloff, Emanuel, 150, 157, 164
second nature, 2, 12–16, 18–19, 22
self-respect, 42–43, 54
socio-cultural, 5, 91, 111–113, 115–117, 141
Statman, Daniel, 42
Stern, William, 2–3, 24, 26–27, 29–30, 33–35
stroke, 4, 92–94
storylines, 5, 97, 99, 176, 183–185, 187, 192
storytelling, 2, 5, 7, 64, 86, 103, 140–141, 151
symptom, 4, 56, 61, 97, 102, 104, 108, 121, 174, 180, 193, 204

Tadd, Winifred, 46
therapeutic emplotment, 96
Thomson, Judith Jarvis, 20
Trebus Project, 85

Universal Declaration of Human Rights, 44, 47

Walker, Margaret Urban, 17
Weber, Max, 13
wisdom, 3, 12, 49–51
Wittgenstein, Ludwig, 16–17